· NO MORE ·
DEPRESSION OR ANXIETY

*End Depression or Anxiety
in as Little as 90 Days*

GARY NULL, Ph.D.

New Longevity Media

©2011 Gary Null.

All rights reserved.

No part of this book may be used or reproduced, stored in a retrieval system or transmitted in any form, or by any means, electronic, mechanical, photocopied, recorded or otherwise, without written permission of the publisher except in the case of brief quotations embodied in critical articles and reviews.

Published by New Longevity Media
www.newlongevitymedia.com

ISBN: 978-0-9835340-1-3, Trade Paperback

Cover design: Lauren Fontaine
Book editor/design: Rachel Trusheim
Copyeditor: Ashley Cadwell

Library of Congress Cataloging-in-Publication Data is available.

The materials presented in this book are designed to present information in support of a healthy lifestyle, but do not guarantee a life free of depression or anxiety. The information is presented for educational purposes only and is not intended to diagnose or treat illness, disease, or any other medical condition. Before acting on any of the information contained in *No More Depression or Anxiety*, the reader agrees that it is his or her sole responsibility to consult with a licensed medical professional (a) to determine whether such information is suitable for the reader; (b) to review any special health concerns, risk factors, or medical conditions, especially if the reader is pregnant or lactating; and (c) to determine whether each of the foods, phytochemicals, supplements, nutrients, herbs, products, appliances, physical exercises, or other actions recommended or presented is appropriate in the specified amounts or is contraindicated for the reader based on any medications that the reader is taking or any other cause or condition relating to the reader, as may be stated in the most recent version of *Physicians' Desk Reference* or other applicable medical authority.

10 9 8 7 6 5 4 3 2 1

Printed in the United States of America.

• TABLE OF CONTENTS •

Introduction		*i*
Chapter 1.	Reexamining the True Nature of Depression and Anxiety	1
Chapter 2.	The Problem with Diagnosis	15
Chapter 3.	Pathologizing Life	21
Chapter 4.	Side Effects of Drugs	50
Chapter 5.	Alternative Treatments for the Body, Nutrition, and Diet	65
Chapter 6.	Comparing Orthodox Versus Alternative Therapies and Their Outcomes	80
Chapter 7.	Positive Affirmations	110
Chapter 8.	Mood-Altering Recipes	147
Chapter 9.	Love	190
Chapter 10.	Experts Speak Out	195
Chapter 11.	Testimonials	219
Chapter 12.	Conclusion	237
Appendix for Alternative Health Studies		*240*
References		*267*

· INTRODUCTION ·

Today it would be easier to ask who is not depressed than who is. After all, look at the environment we live in.

People are anxious or depressed about the effects of an unstable economy. We have approximately six million millionaires, mostly upper mobile baby boomers. That seems great. But we also have more than 60 million people who are living at or below the level of lower middle class who have less disposable income today than they had 25 years ago. A staggering 48 million people are living below the poverty line as we speak. Look at the total amount of people who are on food stamps, unemployed, underemployed, or part-time workers, those who have stopped looking for work, those who are in risk of losing their home to foreclosure (and those who already have), those who are living with relatives or are homeless, and the millions of students who would have gone from college into the workforce but are instead going back home. Add to that all the people who should have been gainfully employed but had to move back home in their 40s and 50s. Think of all the senior citizens who cannot have any quality of life because of the cost of medication, utilities, rent and mortgage, taxes and insurance, and food. Some have no pension and a diminishing Social Security check. And it's not enough to survive. Think of the people who have cancer, heart disease, stroke, and diabetes. Also include those individuals in their 40s, 50s, and 60s now having to take care of their parents, who are now suffering from Alzheimer's and dementia. Think of the increases of crime in neighborhoods that used to be safe. Now in 2011, we are witnessing the ghettoization of the suburbs. There are a million and a half gang members, and the number is growing every day. And think of the people living in areas no longer sustainable due to drought and water shortages, like the areas of Texas, Nevada, California, New Mexico, Arizona, and Utah. Gee, it's a wonder why people go through depressed times.

Unlike our heartier parents and great grandparents who lived through the Depression, we have not been prepared to deal with this. We have an entire generation not competent in geography, philosophy, civics, economics, history, or human relationships. A whole generation who spends up to nine hours a day with their minds and eyes glued to a keypad, Tweeting or engaged to the Internet, and developing virtually no survival skills. These same young people believe that they are perfect and that they deserve everything for just showing up. I wonder if anything can go wrong there. Students are tutored and cram in order to pass a test but are frequently unable to experience real learning. And let's not forget the larger society where our major priority has been competing for who's got the most stuff. Governments, Democrat and Republican, are both corporatist or incapable of serving the real and authentic needs of their constituents. And while all this corruption and malfeasance has been very well disguised in the past, in the present many of our most imminent institutions have betrayed us and go through screaming matches, while none take responsibility for the mistakes they have made. People are outraged at all of the people in power and yet they feel helpless and withdraw into apathy. First comes anger, then comes rage, then comes surrender, and then comes depression. So, of course, I have to ask again. Is there any possible reason people might feel depressed?

Introduction

The middle class was told that, as long as they worked for one company and they did their work correctly, they would receive security, lifetime employment, and wage increases that would have allowed them to have a quality of life for their family. Well it actually worked pretty well through the 1950s, '60s, '70s, '80s, and then we hit a bump, and nothing has been the same since.

Imagine how all of this could impact the youth of today. How do you think they must feel taking out loans for their education only to see the job market diminish before they even get into it? No one knew what credit default swaps and derivatives were or what all those other eloquent Wall Street terms meant, yet we were all affected by it. With the nonstop reporting of the economic recession and Wall Street's careless gambles that constantly threaten our economic stability, it can feel downright impossible to succeed some days.

Think of all the corporations that have merged and the millions of workers who have been fired over the last 30 years due to equity partnerships, buying properties, and then downsizing to make more profit. Michael Milkin, T. Boone Pickens, and Carl Icahn were the architects of this disastrous policy, the middle class were the victims who were not emotionally prepared for this, and as a result we are seeing adults of all ages having to start their life all over again. They are moving from their hometowns—places where they felt secure. Leaving friends and family and those things that were important and familiar to them. Erasing from their consciousness all of those thoughts of a permanent home, neighborhood, a job, and security and going wherever they could find work. Every American child should read John Steinbeck's *Grapes of Wrath* to learn about the last great migration that was forced upon middle-class Americans in the 1930s. Corporate mergers have caused the displacement of more than 20 million American middle-class workers. These people were not emotionally prepared for this.

And think of today's grandparents, who are not having an easy time either. In fact, for many senior citizens in our society, it is especially difficult. Many elders, who have painstakingly saved all their working lives for their golden years, have seen their retirements wiped out or substantially reduced, with their 401Ks down about 25 percent on average. Who would have thought that we would no longer be able to take our safety and security and happiness for granted?

Another major issue is our health. With the passage of time, energetic twentysomethings, who focused mostly on dating, marriage, family, career advancement, and a better standard of living, have become 40- and 50-year-olds confronted with a new set of issues including any number of major diseases. People who once took their well-being for granted now find themselves overweight, fatigued, and suffering from insomnia, mood swings, hot flashes, impotency, arthritis, diabetes, high blood pressure, cancer, and a myriad of other diseases, which are the result of years of stress, poor lifestyle, and an inadequate diet.

Americans have difficulty growing older. All things end; everything has an expiration date. But rarely are we prepared for the transitions we must face throughout life and, ultimately, at its end. We are not taught or counseled on how to deal with divorce, or separation, or loss of a loved one, a job, a neighborhood, or our environment. The assumption is you'll know how to deal with it when it comes. The trouble is that is not true.

Frequently once children are grown and gone, parents begin to feel disconnected from a focus that once held meaning and purpose: the empty-nest syndrome. When we have lost loved ones, either through children leaving the nest, divorce, or death, we don't have a way to properly cope. Nor do we know how to approach the unavoidable conclusion of our lives; death is a taboo subject in our youth-oriented society.

Millions of seniors are leading lives of quiet

Introduction

desperation—sitting at home watching television, the phone seldom ringing, many of them distracting themselves until the inevitable happens. At that point of the process if you're an average person, you're left with your memories to sit and drift into melancholy and depression, especially when you reflect on times when you were vital and had passion. When younger we rarely think of it, but then we reach the day in our lives when we become obsolete in the mind of today's sped-up, youth-driven society. We become irrelevant. We are too old, and we don't have the looks or the physique or the sharp mind that society demands in order to keep our moment in the spotlight. We are reminded through commercials and programming, move on, you've had your day, let us have our time in the sun. Go live in your gated community in Scottsdale, Arizona, Naples, Florida, or Palm Beach, Florida. Hang out with people your own age, whose route is not ahead, since we all fear the inevitable bump we're soon going over. Resign to sameness, blandness. Watch television and read the newspaper and its obituaries. And if you forget your place, there are commercials to remind you that you're the ones they want to sell hemorrhoid cream, osteoporosis drugs, plastic surgery, funeral plots, AARP memberships, and Viagra.

Gee, I wonder, could that type of discrimination and alienation be a cause for mood swings and depression? Remember, we don't expect the seniors who have lived full lives to suffer despair, and there are those who are living happily, but they are a minority compared to those who are indebted (over a trillion dollars a year, collectively) in medical expenses. Feeling neglected, sick, and tired, our elders simply ask, what is the point of it anyways? When was the last time we looked at suicide rates in seniors? They're very high, along with their rates of alcohol and drug abuse.

There is a pervading atmosphere of despair in our fast-paced world today that has not been seen since the 12 years of the Great Depression. Not only did the people suffer no social services for most of that time, but then they went right into the Second World War. That's 16 years of hardship. They were frugal plus strong in mind and character. They saved, adapted, and suffered but survived. That is why they are known as the Greatest Generation.

In contrast, think of a career woman today: a woman in her 30s with a college degree and family. Imagine the pressure of multitasking, of trying to fit everything in some priority of importance in a day's schedule. Think of the stress that is created from trying to get her child into the right preschool, kindergarten, and elementary school. Think of her guilt of not spending quality time with her child or partner but rather enlisting other people to be guardians while she's busy at the workplace. There is little time for the things that make life worthwhile—reading a good book, a special hobby, enjoying cultural events, a quality relationship, quiet downtime, candlelit dinners, bubble baths, long walks in the park, a jog on the beach, or dancing. Nice thoughts, but they are rarely accomplished. More often than not, it's what we hope to get done when we get to that special place of security, however, it rarely happens. As a result, we get chronic anxiety. We are trying to please and be responsible for too many people and too many projects at the same time. We try to master the art of juggling, but then the balls begin to drop and land like lead on our feet. Instead of changing the circumstance that precipitates this excessive, hyperkinetic lifestyle, we simply distract our pain and anxiety and depression with sublimations like overeating, drinking alcohol, drugs, tranquilizers, exercise, shopping, gambling, or Facebook. These are all part of the art of distraction.

How common is it to find people within the American workforce who say that they are happy with their environment and themselves and who say they are achieving the things they have wanted to in a way that gives them a quality of life rather than just a standard of living? In today's competitive society, men and women are not encouraged to cooperate as much as they are forced to compete. They so often look at everyone else as the hostile other. This need to compete challenges people to work harder, to do more, to get ahead and stay ahead, as if all the advantages are somewhere in front of them, and they just haven't worked hard enough or are smart enough to grasp them. And if you have, the moment you stop working, someone else is standing behind you, ready to take it from you. This cycle burns people out.

To dissipate feelings of anxiety, some people turn to exercise. Interestingly, when I go to the gym, I see a lot of people working out, but they do not have happy faces. What I see is a heightened intensity, as if people there are burning off stress. When I go to the gym at noon, I see packed yoga classes. But even this is a vigorous, sweat-producing activity. After class, they are rushing back frequently to a toxic and overly stimulating environment. They think of that one hour of yoga as just enough to sublimate the anxiety they are feeling. The gym today is not the environment for socializing that it was in the 1970s. Rather, it's almost opening a vein on a treadmill to release the toxins of the day.

Their coworkers, on the other hand, may be drinking at a bar to create a buzz that takes the edge off. Or maybe they're smoking marijuana. More Americans are anesthetizing themselves now than ever before. And yes, it will take the pain away for a moment. But we also now have evidence that it can induce paranoia, delusional psychoses, and extreme anxiety and depression. When the anxiety or depression comes back after withdrawal from the drug, the only way to get over it is to go back on the drug again, creating perpetual, long-term abuse.

Other people will sublimate their anxiety by overeating. They don't really care what their bodies look like and will sit in front of a television set, drink beer, and eat pizza and fried chicken. Women will commiserate with Oprah and Dr. Phil, their favorite soap operas, and weepy movies where they identify, "Yes, I'm crying with you because my life is something of a reflection." Most men still believe that a real man doesn't cry and show his feelings, and they displace their feelings by watching sports on television, or working on a car, or going bowling. These are not bad outlets but rather one way of taking the edge off their anxiety and depression.

Today in 2011, we have five million American homes that have been foreclosed. Another six million are underwater in the Gulf of Mexico and will probably be foreclosed. Now 50 million people are on food stamps. The middle class, the working class, and the poor are living with chronic anxiety. That's more than 200 million people.

So, take a look around. See the political and economic instability in the world in which we live, the disintegration of the American family, and people working too hard with inadequate support systems. When we look at the circumstances that are beyond our capacity to manage, we should not wonder why so many Americans feel depressed and anxious.

Another part of the problem in our society is that abnormal life circumstances are viewed as normal situations. We are expected to adjust to them, and if we can't, the fault lies within us, we're told. This way of thinking was prompted several years ago by Eli Lilly for Prozac. Lilly tried to make it seem as if depression was the result of a brain chemical imbalance and that by taking their drug we would feel better and resolve the problem. The idea caught on and other conditions were attributed to this imbalance. If a woman had PMS, her brain was imbalanced. If a child asked too many questions or got up from his seat in the classroom too many times, he was told that he had a brain chemical imbalance.

Today we've made being a child into a disease and millions of children are labeled with ADD, ADHD, and other acronyms. In this generation alone we have 10 million children on prescription medications each day for the control of their behavior. When I was growing up, you never saw any child ever being medicated for such a reason. When you had problems, you talked about them with your family over dinner. If there was the need for outside counseling, you generally would speak with your favorite schoolteacher or Sunday school teacher, rabbi, priest, or minister. Or an aunt, uncle, or grandparent. Only if something were really, really bad you would see a psychologist, and that was rarely talked about. It merely happened. Most of the time you were able to understand the problem and work through it. That did not mean that everything was good again, or that everything was going to get better, but at least you were able to cope. Today it is the exception to be asked questions to get to the root of the problem.

There is a great amount of evidence showing the negative effects various substances have on the brain's chemistry and how the use of even prescribed medications affects a person's mood. Hence, we can artificially create depression or anxiety symptoms by such things as refined sugars, the artificial chemicals added to processed foods, pesticides, milk products, antibiotics, birth control pills, and a hundred of other commonly consumed products. An irony of ironies, the very drugs purported to help these so called "ADD" and "ADHD" children may negatively alter brain chemistry and result in depression and anxiety.

Also, you can have medical conditions that have depression or anxiety as a side effect. Often, they go undiagnosed. For example, a person goes to a doctor complaining of black moods. The patient is fatigued and overweight, and the doctor prescribes an antidepressant when, in fact, it might have been an underactive thyroid gland (three symptoms of an underactive thyroid gland are depression, fatigue, and being overweight). Or the person might be hyperglycemic. Rather than check the blood sugar, the doctor may only look at the symptoms and diagnose depression. An antidepressant is prescribed when the cause of the depression, an erratic blood sugar level, could have been easily corrected with a simple diet change and supplements. What if a child is allergic to milk, and the allergy manifests in the brain and causes hyperactivity? Or anxiety? I can assure you that the doctor, psychologist, or schoolteacher is not going to tell little Jimmy, "Let's check to see if brain allergies are manifesting as a hyperactive reaction to something you have eaten or drank." No, they're going to say, "Jimmy's ADHD and needs Ritalin." So, our society has taken the cue from the pharmaceutical industry, a compliant medical industry, and a teaching profession that purports that all of the symptoms of depression and anxiety are real brain abnormalities that require medical attention and drugging. This is unfortunate because it has made us dependent. In effect, it has made us beholden to most (but not all) of the psychologists, psychiatrists, primary physicians, pediatricians, and schoolteachers to tell us what to do, and they are all singing from the same drug songbook.

Of course, nothing changes as the conditions that led to these feelings go unresolved. And often we have worse feelings. People who would have never thought of suicide, after taking certain medications, including children, now think of suicide. It's an effect of psychotropic medications. Children who are not truly depressed frequently become depressed as one of the effects of antidepressants.

Have the safety and efficacy of these medications been challenged? No. Have any of the true underlying causes of the conditions been looked at? Not often enough. Massive PR campaigns back up physicians who prescribe these medications and the pharmaceutical industry who creates these drugs and the notion that we need them. The National Institute of Mental Health unquestioningly supports them.

Introduction

Nobody wants to take the responsibility for having been wrong. As the legal and political consequences are great, everyone is in denial and nothing gets better.

This book will examine the real causes of our troubles, especially the problem of everyone thinking they're depressed or anxious and in need of a medical fix. If I were writing this book 15 years ago, I might have started with a good diet and proper supplementation and ended with exercise and stress management, but today is a different time and requires a different approach. Also, we have a new, younger generation that feels that they are uniquely susceptible to anxiety and depression.

Hence, we have not examined how we have managed in just a 15-year period to virtually pathologize life. No one is safe from being considered to have a disease that needs to be treated with the appropriate drugs or hospitalization. African Americans, senior citizens, women, and children have been especially susceptible to the pharmaceutical industry's drugging campaigns. I have therefore written an extended chapter showing how we have abused tens of millions of people over the decades without the media, social leaders, even activists being aware of what was happening. If we are to correct the problem, we have to face it, and a pill is not the only answer.

Today if you are an independent nonconformist you can be diagnosed according to the *Diagnostic and Statistical Manual of Mental Disorders (DSM-IV)* as having "oppositional deficit disorder." Hence, any mood or behavior can be pathologized.

I then ask a simple question. Is your medical diagnosis accurate? It has taken me a long time to review the scientific literature to show that across the board, in every single area of medicine, major frauds are being perpetrated. Therefore, to rely solely on the judgment of your primary care physician could be a fatal mistake. The information here could save you from becoming yet another iatrogenic (medical error) statistic. Think of the millions of American women receiving synthetic hormone replacement therapy for their hot flashes and night sweats, who are now shown to have high incidence of heart disease, cervical cancer, dementia, stroke, colorectal cancer, and breast cancer because of their synthetic hormone medicine.

At the other end, I will present scientific literature that supports the use of alternative, natural, nontoxic approaches for dealing with anxiety and depression. We will look at various approaches as we explore guided imagery, neurolinguistic programming, therapeutic touch, tai chi, qigong, homeopathy, Bach flower remedies, intravenous vitamin drips, detoxification, supplementation, and holistic psychotherapy.

Your primary care doctor or psychiatrist will not tell you about S-adenosylmethionine, known as SAMe, a natural substance that is crucial to virtually every cell in the body. It is a simple combination of the essential amino acid methionine and adenosine triphosphate (ATP), which is important as an energy molecule in all living cells. ATP gives needed carbon to certain proteins, fats, RNA, and DNA. When SAMe donates carbons, it keeps transmitters in the brain at an optimal level. It also helps the fat that makes up nerve cell membranes to function in a way that allows the nerves to work properly. Many people walk around with low grades of blue moods. Medicine has given this a name: subsyndronal depression, or intermittent recurrent minor depression. This is just a blue mood that 400–500 milligrams of SAMe can in many cases effectively overcome. It also works faster than antidepressants without side effects. (The only person who shouldn't take it is a manic-depressive who is on other medications. You don't want to go off the medications by yourself, as that can be dangerous.)

There is also something as simple as realizing that from Thanksgiving through Christmas until springtime, people frequently feel sad. They lose their energy, have difficulty

Introduction

waking in the morning, crave sweets and starches, gain weight, and withdraw from friends. They have a difficult time concentrating or working. Why? SAD, or seasonal affective disorder. In the northern states it's especially bad, and in Florida and Southern California it's not seen as often. The reason is a lack of sunlight. To treat SAD, a simple natural protocol of using sunlight can make a big difference.

We will also discuss the benefits of methylation, the simple transfer of a methyl group, which is a molecule made up of one part carbon, three parts hydrogen, that travels around the body causing reactions. This transfer is what happens when we detoxify harmful chemicals from the body. Methylation is related to the melatonin and serotonin cycle, and it relates to mood. There are different nutrients in enhanced methylation, like dimethylglycine (DMG) and SAMe. There are a variety of studies showing that SAMe helps with depression and helps with methylation.

Also, to prove that we must approach this problem from a holistic point of view, I will discuss in depth an antidepression, antianxiety study I did with three groups of people. In one group, people were given advice on a holistic diet, lifestyle, stress management, and behavior modification for dealing with problems in life, plus exercise. In another group, people were just given brain nutrients, ones known to enhance mood, like melatonin, a special form of tryptophan, and coenzyme Q10. In yet another group, these two approaches were combined and people received both the nutrients and the lifestyle recommendations. In this group, there were tremendous changes. People who had been clinically depressed for 30 years overcame their depression in three months. Clearly, if true brain chemical imbalances were causing depression and anxiety, a lifestyle change would not have made a difference, but it did, proving that these are not chemical imbalances but merely ways we can enhance our sense of well-being. This is a far better approach for people to take than the current medical model.

In the next chapters of the book, I'll present wonderful recipes to bring nutritious, energizing, cleansing foods back into our diets. In this section, there is great variety from which to choose and meals that can be made with joy and ease. Whether you are 16 or 60, this should be an important part of the program.

Plus, I found many who were depressed or anxious also had defective immune systems. Indeed, in many a side effect of depression is an immune system that plummets, making us more susceptible to diseases of all types. I have therefore included a section on ways to enhance your immune system. Here you will find ways to build your immune system and keep it strong.

Finally, I have listed positive affirmations. These are my own original affirmations that I have used within my study group. I ask that you take one affirmation per day and focus on it.

In essence, this book is different from others on this subject. It deals with issues that the depressed or anxious person may not have ever thought of before, but it is one that can save your life, or certainly save you from the harm of being misdiagnosed, misprescribed, or mistreated.

The following is an outline of the *Seven Steps to Eliminating Depression and Anxiety Disorders*. Be aware that success in this program requires that a lifestyle modification take place. A lifestyle modification, as the term implies, involves real change. And I can't emphasize strongly enough that this change may be uncomfortable, especially if the practices involved are radically new and different from your current way of life and require frequent daily reminders. In most cases, discomfort should be expected to some degree. If you can get past your "comfort zone," then the results are guaranteed to change your life for the better, but not for good unless you maintain this new approach to life. For example, if you eat hamburgers, hot dogs, and barbequed chicken and cannot imagine life without this traditional American cookout fare, then you are most likely in a comfort zone. Remember that if you find it hard to say "no" to something, then you are probably well within your comfort zone and should probably evaluate whether that something could have a negative impact on your life. Think of the changes that are being suggested in this book, and if they seem too difficult or uncomfortable and lead to thoughts of delaying the process, then realize the following. The greater the resistance to implementing these steps in your life, the richer and greater the rewards will be in the end. Just as three people who are about to undertake a mountain climbing expedition may each gain different levels of reward from taking the summit and reaching the other side of the mountain, it's the person who had the greatest resistance and desire to climb the mountain that we can objectively say overcame the greatest amount of negativity. And it's this potential of overcoming negativity that is truly valuable in overcoming depression and anxiety disorders. Beyond the purely physical aspects of overcoming this disorder, psychological success, as in achieving a goal, has the potential of releasing regenerative, positive energies that in themselves are pure and healing. And what will their rewards be more specifically? Although they come in many forms, the best possible way to phrase what the outcome of this program is would be to go to the testimonial section of this book. Read about actual changes and the conditions that existed prior to the changes. I'll see you on the other side of the mountain.

Seven Steps to Eliminating Depression and Anxiety Disorders

Step 1: How to Identify and Eliminate Risk Factors

This first step is crucial in determining what foods and other substances might be causing allergic reactions, which may very well be the cause of your depression.

One way to identify risk factors is by using the Coca Pulse Test. In the morning upon arising, without getting out of bed, take your pulse. After you take your pulse, place a food that you would like to test for allergic reactions under your tongue. Wait a few minutes. Now take your pulse again. If your pulse increases more than five beats, it's quite likely you are allergic to that food, and that food should be eliminated from your diet. Foods that should be typically eliminated altogether are: animal products, wheat, all dairy, all processed sugars, hydrogenated oils, nightshade vegetables, and simple carbohydrates like white wheat pasta. Also, note that eating organic foods is very important, since even if you eat a recommended food, if it is loaded with pesticides it will undoubtedly be harmful to you and may cause low-grade or even severe allergic reactions.

Step 2: Cleansing and Detoxifying

Detoxification involves several systems of the body including the liver, the kidneys, the large intestine, skin, lungs, and lymphatic system. Each of these systems can be individually detoxified through various techniques.

Detoxifying the liver, the "workhorse organ," is essential. This can be done through a juice therapy cleanse, whereby you build up to five or six vegetable juices and one fruit juice per day. This cleanse should ideally be scheduled for one week. Meals should be limited to once per day. The balance of your nutrition in this cleanse should come from juices and protein shakes. You can use any quality soy- or rice-based protein powders. This cleanse should be conducted for one continuous week at least two times a year. Several juices should be consumed a day.

During this week of detoxification, perform moderate or light exercise in order to enhance the body's cleansing

Introduction

through perspiration and increased circulation. Saunas or hot baths are also suggested in order to detoxify through the skin. Remember not to exceed more than 15 minutes per sauna session. Always keep well hydrated during heat cleanses. Drink up to one gallon of water or juice per day.

Coffee enemas are also very beneficial for the liver cleanse as well as the large intestine. Organic coffee should be diluted to a light golden color and chilled to room temperature. It can then be administered via an enema, retaining the coffee a total of three minutes. It may be difficult at first to retain the liquid, so here are a few tips. Do a water enema first, using fresh, clean water at room temperature. This does not have to be retained. It can be released as soon as the urge appears. After the water is fully evacuated, you may administer the coffee, retaining the liquid for one minute on your right side, one minute on your back, and finally one minute of your left side. Do not exceed a total of three minutes. Acidophilus and bifidus, the good bacteria, should be consumed after the enema session.

Therapeutic breathing for 15 minutes daily will help relieve stress as well as reteach the body to completely exhale carbon dioxide. This will minimize toxic gaseous buildup in the blood, resulting in increased overall energy and greater oxygen utilization. Following is a cleansing tea that can do wonders. Steep one teaspoon of dried dandelion leaf and one teaspoon marshmallow root in a cup of boiling water. Strain, let cool, and drink with stevia or honey. You may repeat this five times daily. This drink is rich in minerals such as potassium. Herbs have been frequently used in cleansing. Dandelion leaf promotes diuresis. Corn silk soothes urinary tract inflammation. The herb bearberry (uva-ursi) has been associated with relieving bladder stone pains and bedwetting.

Red clover is an excellent herb for lymphatic detoxification as well as echinacea and gingko biloba.

One of the best ways to help cleanse the lymphatic system

is through exercise, especially rebounding and more high-impact routines. If joint problems are a concern, exercises such as low-impact aerobics and more vigorous forms of yoga may be useful as well.

Step 3: Rejuvenation

Now that you've cleansed your body internally, it's time to incorporate proper nutrients to rejuvenate the integrity of your cells. Remember, it's important to detoxify prior to beginning the nutritional protocol because most of the nutrients that you consume will be assimilated in the large intestine. Please review the anxiety and depression protocols recommended later in this book. Begin by taking the supplements one at a time and building recommended dosages slowly as well.

Step 4: De-Stressing Our Lives

A major contributor to all the killer diseases is stress. Stress exacerbates most maladies and reduces the immune system, making the body susceptible to the occurrence of factors that contribute to an array of other conditions. This is why the mother of all diseases can most certainly be called "stress."

So what can a person do to control this killer? First of all, it's important to note stress in and of itself can be useful. It's ultimately the way stressful situations are perceived in one's life that can make all the difference. For example, consider two people who have to give a public speech. One individual is confident and enjoys speaking, while the other is more reserved, shy, and fearful of saying the wrong thing. They both have the same task at hand, yet the individual who is fearful will produce cortisol, a biochemical associated with the development of heart disease. Recurrences of similarly stressful situations in that person's life could ultimately lead to the development of depression as well.

There are many approaches that can be taken in reducing

negative reactions to stressful situations. One, for example, is prayer. Many studies have been conducted on the power of prayer. You need not be religious in order to speak to a higher power. Just acknowledging a higher power that may guide one's life could be a relief in and of itself. Letting go of the ego and allowing your image of a higher power show you the next obstacle, hurdle, or challenge is a refreshing viewpoint to begin with. Asking that higher power for guidance with absolute faith that you are being listened to can displace your dependence from wanting to be in control. Only then will it be possible to innately listen for direction.

Other methods of stress management are meditation, qigong, tai chi, yoga, herbs (valerian skull cap herb, St. John's wort, lemon balm, and chamomile), and nutrients (GABA and threonine) are very useful too. I can't emphasize strongly enough that you must choose some form of stress management on a regular basis, and you stick with it. The more you practice, the better you feel and releasing stress will become second nature. I've created a series of videos and audiotapes that address self-empowerment and stress management issues. These are helpful tools that introduce fresh perspectives on how to manage stress by shifting your entire paradigm so that you can recognize yourself and your true roles in life, while maintaining a compassionate heart for all.

Step 5: Removing Toxins from Personal and Home Environment

Go through your home and take inventory of all potential environmental toxins. Toxins can be found in places you don't even expect. Dust and mold has to be reduced or eliminated because they could cause severe immune responses resulting in disease. You must replace chemical-laden toothpastes, cosmetics, and mouthwashes with natural products. Eliminate the use of fluoride. Shop for organic, whole foods. Even the garments you wear should be considered. It's best to wear or

NO MORE DEPRESSION OR ANXIETY

use bedding that is made of cotton, silk, and other natural fibers. These fibers should ideally be untreated by chemicals. Buy a quality air and water purification unit. Never drink tap water. These are just a few recommendations. Outline the variables that compose your environment and research the constituents. This approach will prepare you to always question environmental surroundings and avoid personal environmental toxicity for life.

Step 6: Exercise

It is common knowledge these days that exercise is important for optimal health. But what kind of exercise, and how frequently should it be done? When considering exercise, we must consider movements that benefit our cardiovascular system and lymphatic system as well as overall muscular strength and endurance. Aerobic exercise in all its forms will typically address cardiovascular improvements as well as improve lymphatic stimulation.

Though the choices of aerobic exercise may vary greatly, and include activities such as running, power walking, swimming, bicycling, cross-country skiing, floor aerobics, tae bo, using aerobic machines such as Stairmasters or VersaClimbers, and the list goes on. The formula for ensuring that your aerobic work is optimally effective is as follows. Aerobic exercise should begin at 10 to 20 minutes, five days a week and built up to approximately 45 to 60 minutes, five days a week.

Keeping your heart rate in an aerobic zone is the key to proper aerobic conditioning. The aerobic zone is the optimal beats your heart makes per minute, sustained over the course of your workout. For example, your resting heart rate might be 70 beats per minute, but during your workout, the heart should increase to a suitable level for your age.

To find your target heart rate, subtract your age from

the number 220. This will give you your maximal heart rate. Now calculate 75 percent of your maximal heart rate, and that result will be your average target heart rate. For senior citizens or individuals who are overweight by at least 20 pounds, the percentage that should be calculated is 65 percent. Athletes can calculate 85 to 90 percent. For example, a senior citizen who is 70 years old would calculate the following: $220 - 70 = 150$, 150×65 percent $= 97.5$, or rounded up to 98 beats per minute. Now if the senior citizen being discussed is in good shape, he or she may calculate 75 percent of the maximal heart rate. So this senior citizen should exercise aerobically for 45 to 60 minutes maintaining a heart rate of 98 beats per minute for the majority of the work out. This would be a healthy aerobic workout.

Strength training is also important. Again, there are a variety of exercises to choose from, like calisthenics to pilates, but probably the most effective and easily applicable technique is weight training. There are many good books and videos on weight training that would go into more detail than I wish to dedicate in this book. So do your research, and if there's one important tip that I can give about weight training is that whatever you do, maintain proper posture and fluid breathing in whatever exercise you choose. And even though you must work at a good intensity, enough to eventually break into a sweat, always remember: train, don't strain!

Step 7: No More Excuses

As I mentioned earlier in this chapter, reaching beyond your "comfort zone" is probably the single most important concept that needs to be understood and applied in order to maintain the lifestyle modifications that I am suggesting. Every day, all that we do is just a series of choices. We have the ability to choose what is good and positive in every moment.

If this is so, then why don't we always choose what is good and positive but instead frequently settle on choices that are ultimately self-destructive? This is the "comfort zone" that I am referring to.

It is quite possible that because of your conditioning, which typically comes from your upbringing and other similar factors, your "comfortable" choices, the ones that you've been accustomed to, are not quite the best ones for your optimal health, friendships, love relationships, and even your finances. Identifying where you have a certain "rub" or "discomfort" is the first step to releasing yourself from the cycle you are in. Remember: the mind that caused the problem can never be the mind that solves the problem. So in order to switch from the mind that created the problem to one that can solve it undoubtedly requires a sensation of "discomfort."

The very first thought and place to begin is "No More Excuses." What this means is that you must begin to assertively seek out all conditions and cycles in your life that don't contribute to your optimal well-being and the joy of sharing that you can experience among other people. Don't allow an excuse to get in your way of starting on the right track. I don't have enough money, or I don't have enough time, or I'll start next week (which usually means never), or I can't do it alone, and the list can go on as long as there are excuses. But what if you didn't allow for any excuses? What if that was a possibility? Well then what? You WILL succeed at this program AND any other task you wish to undertake in your life. It's so easy and comfortable to procrastinate, so reach out, without any excuses, for the great potential that you innately have.

• CHAPTER 1 •

Reexamining the True Nature of Depression

There is an incredible increase in the number of people who are suffering from anxiety and depression. Instead of studying the real reasons for this increase, the pharmaceutical industry, with the support of doctors, HMOs, and primary care physicians, seems to think it has the answer to the problem of anxiety and depression in the form of a pill. But what can we learn from studying the history of depression? There was a time when depression was categorized as mental illness causing the patient to be shunned from society. Even into the 1970s people would be reluctant to admit to seeing a psychiatrist or taking antidepressant medication. We used to have human services where real people counseled face-to-face others who had psychological imbalance. Part of the rise in the field of psychiatry itself may stem from people having less interaction with older, wiser relatives and friends. When our days are so congested with the responsibilities of work and family, we barely have time to talk to our own partner or children. We hire psychologists to perform the service of a kindly aunt or uncle. But they are letting us down and spending less and less time in talk therapy. And with the advent of psychiatric medication for anxiety and depression, much of the talk therapy was put aside and drug therapy became the treatment. Mental illness was defined as either a brain disorder or a chemical imbalance, with the end result of applying a drug to a particular diagnosis.

Whereas infectious diseases are said to be the result of external germs invading the physical body, mental illness is thought to be something that develops from a problem within the brain or within brain chemistry. This is an interesting twist on the mind-body separation in allopathic medicine. The physical body is under assault from the external environment, whereas our brain and body biochemistry are under additional assaults from that which we eat, breathe, and drink. Of course, this is true when the outside world can trigger a stress reaction and set the stage for anxiety and depression.

Once it was found that serotonin was a mood-elevating neurotransmitter, then overnight through a massive propaganda effort, ghostwriters, publicists, and scientists for hire created the myth of serotonin deficiency, which then became the primary diagnosis of what could cause the imbalance that in turn causes depression. Because of the mind-body split, it was not thought possible that a bad diet, nutrient deficiency, or exposure to noxious chemicals could affect the mind. The cause of the chemical imbalance in the brain was not investigated. What was important was that there was a chemical imbalance in the brain that could possibly be treated by drugs. Scientists, engaged in their own unique form of alchemy, had created a drug that was considered the treatment of choice for balancing serotonin. The drug was Prozac.

Even though depression is said to be a chemical imbalance, the diagnosis does not involve measuring the brain chemistry. It's just taken for granted that a serotonin deficiency causes depression. So if a person presents symptoms that resemble depression, they are depressed, and are given antidepressant medications. All the while, a mind-boggling number of causes of those symptoms of depression could be occurring, but doctors are frequently missing the real cause when they primarily treat the symptoms.

The witch's bible of psychiatry, a true psychiatric comic book with no science behind it, a pure piece of psychiatric pornography, is called the *Diagnostic and Statistical Manual of Mental Disorders*, fourth edition (*DSM-IV*) and contains the diagnostic criteria for anxiety and depression. Within this book of myths, virtually every single human emotion and reaction can be pathologized, coded, diagnosed, and treated, as if any of it was real. This is equivalent to endless profits for the pharmaceutical industry. From birth to death, they got you, with a compliant, cult-like medical community willing to obey any dictates as if they were real and legitimate, and based on sound science. Not one of which is true. The list is expanding all the time. Recently, premenstrual syndrome (PMS) was elevated to the status of mental illness. And just in time because once you have the disease, you can now be offered the treatment. Serafem is Prozac disguised as a new treatment for PMS.

Most women know when their period is coming with a little aching in the lower abdomen, some mood change, and a feeling like they need to slow down and relax a bit. But that's not always possible in our overly commercialized and hyper-fast society. We're conditioned to think we can't slow down. If we do for a minute of it, then we'll miss out on being responsible.

We are pulled along in the rat race to the point where we don't have time to go through normal life processes or have time to process our own feelings. Menopause and PMS are both considered diseases today and each have their own medical treatments so they won't "interfere" with our lives. But we forget that our lives are about feelings and interaction and communication. If we don't have time for these normal events and just take medications to suppress feelings, we are living on a very superficial plane of existence.

Children, unfortunately, have been drawn into the drug business as well. They also drink a lot of soda with sugar or artificial sweetener, and eat hot dogs dyed with food coloring and enormous amounts of bread and pastries until they end up with vitamin and mineral deficiencies, all which affect their mental functioning. Outside school they spend their time watching TV, surfing the Internet, playing video games, Tweeting, and even talking on cell phones, and they get antsy and bored. As a result, they cycle through a day with extreme highs and lows. Staying alert to "abnormal" behavior, the teacher and school nurse regularly single out kids that can't pay attention, disrupt the class, or demand attention and send them off to the school psychologist. Usually "problem kids" are put on Ritalin under the guise of wanting them to focus on their schoolwork. But no studies have ever shown that Ritalin improves a child's learning. It controls their behavior enough that they no longer disrupt the class or the teacher's set way of teaching.

Once a child grows up on Ritalin, it's not a huge leap for them to accept antidepressants in their young adult life. In fact this is the first generation to grow up considering it normal behavior to take multiple medications each day before going to school. In fact, many students feel there's something wrong with them if they're not on meds. They have grown up on drugs, and if they find they can't cope with the normal stresses and strains of daily living, they fall easily into the habit of taking a mood-elevating drug.

Twenty-five years ago, major clinical medical texts listed several types of depression: depressive neurosis, reactive depression, involutional melancholia, manic-depressive psychosis, and major affective disorder psychosis. Outside the depressive category altogether was a condition called transient situational disturbance such as death in the family or other major episode of grief. Reactive depression was also related to reaction with grief. Involutional melancholia was the term used for a form of depression that sets in after middle age. Major affective disorder psychosis was the name given to depression occurring for no known cause.

Presently, depression is categorized as major depression, dysthymia, and bipolar. According to the National Institutes of Health, major depression is diagnosed when a person has many of the following list of symptoms interfering with the ability to work, study, sleep, eat, and enjoy life:

a. Persistent sad, anxious, or "empty" mood.

b. Feelings of hopelessness, pessimism.

c. Feelings of guilt, worthlessness, helplessness.

d. Loss of interest or pleasure in hobbies and activities that were once enjoyed including sex.

e. Decreased energy, fatigue, being "slowed down."

f. Difficulty concentrating, remembering, or making decisions.

g. Insomnia, early-morning awakening, or oversleeping.

h. Appetite and/or weight loss or overeating and weight gain.

i. Thoughts of death or suicide; suicide attempts.

j. Restlessness, irritability.

k. Persistent physical symptoms that do not respond to treatment such as headaches, digestive disorders, and chronic pain.

Dysthymia is a term that wasn't even in use 25 years ago and greatly widens the definition of depression. It is said to be a less severe type of depression that involves long-term chronic symptoms. These symptoms are not disabling but keep a person from functioning well or from feeling "good." Dysthymia as defined by the American Psychiatric Association and International Classification of Mental Disorders as "a prevalent form of subthreshold depressive pathology and gloominess, anhedonia, low drive and energy, low self-esteem, and pessimistic outlook."

Bipolar disorder is another name for manic depression and defines mood cycles from manic highs to depressive lows. Bipolar is the least common of the three types of depression occurring in 1.2 percent of the population. Major depression occurs in 5 percent and dysthymia in 0.4 percent. In manic-depressives, when depressed, the symptoms of depression manifest; when manic, the following symptoms are found:

a. Abnormal or excessive elation.

b. Unusual irritability.

c. Decreased need for sleep.

d. Grandiose notions.

e. Increased talking.

f. Racing thoughts.

g. Increased sexual desire.

h. Markedly increased energy.

i. Poor judgment.

j. Inappropriate social behavior.

Mania, however, is not the same as anxiety. While depression affects over 40 million American adults, anxiety disorders affect half as many. The anxiety disorders discussed include: panic disorder, obsessive-compulsive disorder, post-traumatic stress disorder, social phobia (or social anxiety disorder), specific phobias, and generalized anxiety disorder (GAD). People with anxiety disorders demonstrate excessive, irrational fear or dread.

The use of drug treatment for anxiety and depression, on the surface, actually suits both patient and doctor. Doctors like it because they think they see fast relief of their patient's symptoms, and they can process more needy patients. Previously, talk therapy might take several hours a week to perform, but once the initial diagnosis was made and a patient put on antidepressant pills, he or she would only have to be seen for a few minutes a month or even every three months to renew the prescription. Some patients love it because they never have to address the reasons why they're depressed. They imagine they have a chemistry imbalance and are treating it with the proper chemical. Also, patients can't afford talk therapy. Talking to a psychiatrist for one or two hours a week can be very expensive compared to a prescription renewal appointment. Some patients resign to the idea that they will never know the real reasons why they're depressed.

Frequently, anxiety and depression have become diagnoses, but really they are a psychological reaction. You may be reacting to losing your job or the death of a family member or having a fight with your partner or children. And yes, this may make you feel down in the dumps, but it doesn't mean you're clinically depressed. You may even say, "I'm depressed," but it's just a term you use to get the point across instead of going into the details.

When psychiatrists define depression they use the *Diagnostic and Statistical Manual of Mental Disorders*, fourth edition (*DSM-IV*). They are very serious about diagnosing depression and categorizing your symptoms because once you are in a particular box, your diagnosis can be matched with an "appropriate" drug. So, perhaps, we are talking about two types of depression, which are becoming interchangeable. The ups and downs of everyday existence are being swept into the psychiatric definition of severe depression.

Along with the ups and downs of everyday existence are the ups and downs of normal neurotransmitters and natural chemicals in the body. In the 1980s depression was equated with the deficiency of the neurotransmitter serotonin in the body. Immediately, pharmaceutical companies sought out a drug that would elevate serotonin levels. What they didn't do was try to find the reasons why. They didn't look at normal body chemistry; they didn't investigate the vitamins, minerals, amino acids, and essential fatty acids—nutrients responsible for creating serotonin in the first place.

When you look at anxiety and depression from a whole-body perspective you see that it can be triggered in dozens of ways. Chemical imbalance of neurotransmitters can be caused by too much sugar in the diet, wheat/gluten allergy, mold allergy, excess alcohol intake, vitamin deficiency, mineral deficiency, essential fatty acid deficiency, amino acid deficiency, chemical allergies (additive and colorings), exposure to toxic chemicals and heavy metals, and side effects of almost any prescription medication. But when the sole treatment for chemical imbalance is thought to be synthetic drugs, we lose sight of the delicate biochemistry of the mind and the body, which can be manipulated by food and other medications.

What are we to make of a recent study, which showed that a placebo was even more effective in helping people with depression than Prozac? There are several aspects to consider. It certainly makes you wonder whether the drug is doing anything positive at all. If the placebo works better, then the drug was actually making people feel worse. Also the study showed that there were brain chemistry changes attributable to the placebo identical to the changes with the drug. But what they are forgetting is that anyone who takes the pill, whether placebo or medication, is going to have a placebo effect.

The placebo effect occurs when a person's own healing mechanisms are triggered. Thinking that you are taking a pill that will help you stimulate you to help yourself. Modern medicine has forgotten that the most important aspect of treating patients is to develop a rapport and let the patients know you want to help them. With the rise of HMOs and the mechanization of medicine, doctors are only given minutes to spend with a patient and increasingly have become drug prescribers. They no longer have quality time to get to know their patients. Knowing about someone's job, family, diet, and goals are very important ways of connecting with the patient and also help the doctor connect the dots to a correct diagnosis. If your doctor knows that you work in a toxic environment, it can help him or her decide whether you are suffering irritability and depression due to toxic chemicals. Knowing that you drink 10 cups of coffee a day can certainly help your doctor decide that's what may be triggering your heart palpitations and feelings of anxiety. Knowing your father just died after a lengthy illness can help your doctor decide you're going through a normal grieving process superimposed on exhaustion for which you need time off from work, not a drug prescription.

The altruistic medical advisors, like Marcus Welby of the 1960s and Sanjay Gupta today, seem beyond our reach now. Instead, television drug ads make the diagnosis of anything from PMS to heartburn and gastrointestinal problems, to anxiety and depression right on the screen. Drug companies know that people spend most of their free time sitting in front of the television. They also know television puts people in a receptive and suggestible mode. The entertainment content of television also plays a part. The dramas are often violent and depressing and the sitcoms are sugarcoated mini-dramas where all the problems in a family are worked over in a half hour. After a while you become conditioned to think that you too are depressed and that there are easy solutions to your problems. Those solutions are the ads. It would be interesting to do a study to see where TV ads for antidepressants are placed. Are they predominant during sitcoms or dramas? Are they placed nearer to the end of dramas when people feel more burdened with the weight of the problems on the screen and are in need of a quick-fix solution?

When television ads give a list of anxiety or depression symptoms, most people automatically identify with those symptoms. Especially when those symptoms are so generalized they fit the majority of the population. "Are you feeling stressed? Are you losing sleep due to worrying? Do you want help?" Yes, yes, and yes. These ads, according to the drug companies, are having the desired effect of people marching into their doctor's offices demanding medication to make them feel good. And they might feel good initially. Perhaps it's due to the placebo effect, and perhaps because they weren't depressed in the first place. But they think someone listened to them, even for only a short time, and a doctor gave them something to make them feel better.

The placebo effect kicks in and they perk up, for a time. But then, echoing in the background is the rapid-fire list of side effects that the drug companies are required to recite during their commercials. It goes something like: this drug can cause nausea, vomiting, diarrhea, constipation, anaphylactic shock, and symptoms up to, and including, death. In men it's impotence, which has another easy fix. If a man keeps taking the drug because his prescription has refills, his doctor can just write another prescription for Viagra.

Now this man was already taking Tums and Metamucil for the drying effects of the medication that made him feel nauseous and gave him constipation. But what he didn't know was that the calcium carbonate in the antacid tablet was neutralizing his stomach acid, and he wasn't digesting his food properly. Gradually, he became more fatigued and lethargic because he wasn't absorbing the nutrients from undigested food. In order to cope with that, he drank more coffee and ate more sweets. Then he knew he was really depressed and anxious because he began to gain weight and now had heart palpitations. Never once did he realize that these symptoms were all the result of the antacid tablet. Or that he was developing hypoglycemia from the excessive sugar in his diet. Or that he was deficient in magnesium, which can cause heart symptoms. Neither did his doctor know what was really going on; he or she never asked him about their patient's diet but instead prescribed heart medication for the palpitations and an anxiolytic drug for the anxiety.

Viagra in a patient with heart symptoms is a possible contraindication, but the doctor had forgotten he had given his patient a renewable prescription. Each drug that was added was justified in the doctor's chart and approved by the HMO billing codes. However, each drug was adding to the patient's toxicity and putting increasing strain on the liver's capacity to detoxify.

When drug companies list side effects in the *Physicians' Desk Reference* (PDR), they happily do so because if the side effect is listed, then it's difficult to prevail if you sue. They have reported the side effect, and the doctor should at least be aware of what's been reported. But the doctor doesn't necessarily read about every drug he prescribes, and most patients have no idea they could be taking a "time bomb." Even if they are aware of the side effects, some patients feel like it won't happen to them, and others have been made complacent by the amount of drugs in use today. Patients often feel that if a drug has been prescribed by a doctor, then it *must* be safe. They don't realize that almost half of the drugs that reach the market are removed and relabeled within 10 years for dangerous side effects. In the intervening 10 years the number of fatalities and adverse reactions add up.

In the field of nutritional medicine with its common knowledge of dozens of alternatives to drugs, it's hard to imagine how a person can rationalize taking drugs with even a glimmer of side effects. Much less drugs that, by verified reports, cause over 100,000 deaths and 10 million severe reactions annually. What are people thinking? Well maybe they're thinking that someone else should do their thinking for them. They've grown up on Marcus Welby, Dr. Kildare, and *ER* and think doctors are heroes. It's the baby boomer generation that has grown up on wild expectations of a great life. Growing up on drugs, the boomers learned to medicate each stage of life, and now they have the expectation that they will be taken care of in their old age with free medications. Boomers, busy following their "bliss," allowed their children and grandchildren to be put on Ritalin and Prozac. They resent the younger Gen Xers and try to stay on top of their game with Prozac and Viagra.

Doctors, meanwhile, have become disenfranchised from their traditional roots. They've become employees of HMOs, unable to make even the simplest of decisions regarding the welfare of their patients. Most doctors have no awareness of the mind-body connection or that food, drugs, and chemicals can cause depression. But in the current HMO settings with appointment times averaging about seven minutes, there is not even enough time for a friendly interaction with patients that might be reassuring to those undergoing stress. Now they are faced with doctors who are as stressed as they are.

In this book we point out that depression is being vastly overdiagnosed and overmedicated, and alternative therapies are being completely ignored by mainstream medicine. But it gets worse. Even if a doctor knows that anxiety and depression can be caused by hypoglycemia, nutrient deficiencies, or chemical intoxication, he or she may not be allowed to do the appropriate testing to make the proper diagnosis. An HMO clerk can unilaterally make the decision that a particular test for glucose tolerance in an anxious or depressed patient doesn't fall into the criteria of tests that can be ordered for anxiety or depression. He or she cancels the test. Otherwise the patient has to pay out of pocket for the test. If a doctor orders vitamin or mineral blood test for a patient and an HMO clerk doesn't find those tests on the "approved" list the same thing happens—the test is cancelled. If a doctor orders blood tests for heavy metals, thinking that mercury or lead toxicity could play a role in this patient's depression, the test will likely be cancelled.

As long as the prevailing opinion in the medical community is that depression is caused by a serotonin deficiency (even though serotonin is rarely tested in the patient), then any other tests are deemed unnecessary. If a doctor tries to fight for these tests for his patient, he usually wastes his time, or worse, his behavior sets off a red flag at HMO headquarters. Similarly, if a doctor writes letters on a patient's behalf to recover money spent on tests not covered by the patient's insurance, the doctor's billing practices are carefully scrutinized. If the doctor falls outside the "standard practice of medicine" by ordering unapproved tests, using unapproved treatments, or even by prescribing fewer drugs than his peers, he can be brought in front of his state medical board to answer such charges. Health care should largely be the responsibility of the individual, but when doctors are routinely disciplined for avoiding prescribing drugs to their patients, it makes it difficult for patients to find a doctor sympathetic to alternatives. And it means that doctors are never going to be able to make any changes to the system. They are too vulnerable to their medical board; they can lose their license and their livelihood too easily for sticking their heads out.

So, it's up to you, readers. It's up to you to understand the problem we are facing in our health care system. It's up to you to take a stand, to take charge of your health and your health care. To give you ammunition and support for your own healing this book reviews hundreds of studies proving the effectiveness and safety of alternative therapies for anxiety and depression. Start with the basics, a good organic diet, natural supplements, exercise, and simple relaxation techniques, and you'll be amazed at how much better you feel.

• CHAPTER 2 •

The Problem with Diagnosis

The Washington Post ran a series of articles on depression from January to May 2002. In his January 9th article, staff writer Shankar Vedantam reported on a study showing a threefold increase in drug therapy for depression from 1987 to 1997. Vedantam felt that "the sea change probably does not stem from an actual increase in depression." And he made an impressive list for possible causes for the unprecedented rise in medical intervention into the moods and emotions of our population. He said, "instead, it is most likely connected to the de-stigmatization of mental health problems in general and depression in particular, the rise of managed-care insurance plans, and the arrival of powerful drugs including Prozac, accompanied by multi-million dollar marketing campaigns."

It is true that managed health care has effectively systematized mental health care into a primarily drug-based treatment approach, which is much cheaper than extended psychotherapy or hospitalization. Mr. Vedantam reported that about one-third of patients in 1987 were prescribed medications, whereas in 1997 three-quarters were prescribed medications and saw their doctors only two-thirds of the time of the 1987 patients. Treatment also shifted from psychiatrists to primary care physicians and other health care providers. Vedantum said there was a concern by psychiatrists that some of the patients may not be getting the treatment they need and that some might be getting misdiagnosed or overdiagnosed by unqualified people. The psychiatrists, who do more psychotherapy than general practitioners, are concerned not just about patients being mistreated but also about losing their incomes.

In the May 21st *Washington Post* article, Shankar Vedantam again tackled the topic of depression. He said that about 19 million people suffer from depression and almost two-thirds receive no treatment. Depression is being called the most common and most untreated chronic disease. But help is on the way, mostly in the form of drug therapy, from "a top independent advisory panel" that recommends that doctors begin routinely screening all patients for depression and says that "America's primary care doctors are missing and mistreating more than half of all cases of the common mental disorder."

This panel is the government-funded U.S. Preventative Services Task Force, a "highly influential group of scientists that sets widely followed standards on topics ranging from prostate cancer screening to mammograms." Presumably, the panel is not funded by the drug industry, but by investigating their mandate we find that they are all university-based and hospital-based medical doctors. Most university and hospital research is primarily funded by drug companies. So, from all appearances, this panel is going to do nothing more than promote drug therapy for depression. There are all the naturopaths who detoxify and supplement depressed patients, the clinical ecologists who examine brain allergies as a cause of depression, and the certified clinical nutritionists who look at nutritional aspects of depression. When all you have is a hammer, everything looks like a nail. Allopathic medicine has elevated drugs to the status of hammer against the nail of depression.

The Problem with Diagnosis

What's really of concern is the way the task force hopes to swell the ranks of depressed people being treated. They say that every patient should be asked two basic questions on every visit to determine whether they are depressed:

1. "Over the past two weeks, have you felt down, depressed, or hopeless?"
2. "Over the past two weeks, have you felt little interest in doing things?"

The task force advises that if the problems have lasted throughout the previous two weeks and have interfered with the patient's ability to perform day-to-day tasks, doctors may make a diagnosis of depression.

Who hasn't had a time of day when they felt down or received little pleasure in doing things? Does this mean we are all depressed? Maybe that's just the point; maybe we are all supposed to be on Prozac—from a marketing point of view!

What other factors in our environment and culture make us depressed and subject to drug intervention? Let's look at our major forms of cultural entertainment: the Internet, cell phones, movies, and television. For example, Woody Allen and his characterization of "modern man" greatly helped with the de-stigmatization of mental health problems by making everyone feel less neurotic and depressed than he or his characters. He made a visit to the psychiatrist a "normal" event. In the movie *Shampoo,* someone during a panic attack cried out, "Has anyone got a Valium?" followed by a showering of prescription bottles. Now Prozac is the drug du jour. Antianxiety and antidepressant drugs are part of the cultural norm.

Ann Landers, in her popular advice column in 1998, maintained that "80 percent of people with depression are on a combination of the two." In that year she reported there were 17 million depressed Americans. She was an enthusiastic proponent of medical intervention for depression when she reported that on National Depression Screening Day in 1997, more than 85,000 people visited screening sites. She said that for the 1998 National Depression Screening Day on October 8 there would be more than 3,000 free anonymous screening sites all across the country that everyone should attend.

National Depression Screening Day was originated by the National Institute of Mental Health (NIHM), which is part of the United States Department of Health and Human Services, and is now only one of the many sponsors of the program. The program is run by screening for Mental Health, Inc. (SMH, formerly the national Mental Illness Screening Project), "a nonprofit organization developed to coordinate nationwide mental health screening programs and to ensure cooperation, professionalism, and accountability in mental illness screenings." SMH also claims to be involved in several research initiatives that are shedding new light on America's mental health. SMH admits that their programs are supported solely through grants, donations, and registration fees from participating screening sites. Some of their sponsors include: Eli Lilly, Pfizer, Abbott Laboratories, Solvay Pharmaceuticals, Forest Laboratories, GlaxoSmithKline, Organon Increase, and Wyeth Pharmaceuticals.

Eli Lilly makes Prozac for depression, obsessive-compulsive disorder (OCD), bulimia (including long-term treatment), and panic disorder; Sarafem for premenstrual dysphoric disorder (PMDD); and Zyprexa for schizophrenia and acute bipolar mania. Pfizer makes Zoloft and Viagra. These companies provide the educational material and funding for over 3,000 depression testing sites for National Depression Screening Day. A new initiative has installed 500 high schools with depression testing sites.

In 2001 the National Depression Screening Day was mounted "to educate the public about depression and its

The Problem with Diagnosis

symptoms and to encourage individuals to be screened." However, their goals in 2002 were much loftier. They described National Depression Screening Day as "an effort to educate the public nationwide about depression, bipolar disorder (also called manic-depression), anxiety and post-traumatic stress disorder."

Such screening days, under the guise of helping the public deal with the symptoms of depression, may be more about drug companies having access to millions of consumers who may be gullible enough to think that life can be enhanced with a pill.

Yes, the major de-stigmatization of mental health has come from pharmaceutical companies who, according to Mr. Vedantam, offer powerful drugs like Prozac and promote them with million-dollar advertising campaigns, especially on the powerful medium of television. As people sit in front of the TV screen, appearing like couch potatoes, they already have a drug surging through their brains. It's called dopamine. Dopamine creates feelings of alertness, excitement, and aggression. When separated from their TV drug fix, and not knowing they are coming down from a TV high, people feel depressed and they need a drug. They reach for carbohydrates, which increase the levels of serotonin in their brains, and they fill prescriptions for Prozac to revive the "feel-good" sensation.

What did people do in times of great stress in the past? During the First and Second World Wars and in the Great Depression, were people tougher then? Have the privileges of the baby-boomer generation somehow weakened the resolve needed to cope with everyday stresses and everyday emotions without caving in?

Through the years, the increase in anxiety and depression has been blamed on stress. But the obvious fact that we consume more information than previous generations has often been cited as causing stress. We see a horror movie and think we've lived it; our adrenal glands get hammered by the images and adrenaline shoots through our body and speeds up our heart. When it's all over we feel let down. Every time we see a thrilling event on television we go through the same roller coaster, but we have no idea how it's affecting our body chemistry. If it is a horrible world event that we witness, we go through our personal emotions, but then because the media uses these disasters for content to sell advertising, we relive and rehash events over and over until we are exhausted, both physically and mentally. With Lady Diana's death in 1997 and the September 11th tragedy in 2001, armies of reporters and psychiatrists tried to tell us how we were feeling and bathed our raw nerves with more information than we could handle. When you go through an event and it is replayed into your brain a thousand times, we could assume it has a deep impact on your psyche.

There's more afoot than just being brainwashed by TV. Why are people watching so much TV in the first place? Are we a nation where people have just too much time on their hands? The content of a normal brain is worry. But if we busy ourselves with our job, families, and the daily crises that occur, we don't pay much attention to the incessant nagging. The baby boomers with their life-long desires—not to work as hard as their parents, no to be involved in a war, not to work all their lives in a dead-end job that they hate, not to go through another Great Depression—have in fact evoked the opposite. They have created personal depression on a massive scale. They are not content with their lives. And the pharmaceutical companies have marketed this discontent and made them feel that the symptoms can be alleviated by drugs; a mantra reminding us of Soma, the drug given to pacify the population in Orwell's book *1984*.

• CHAPTER 3 •

Pathologizing Life

There is a crisis in the United States today. Forty million of its citizens are diagnosed with depression. An increasing number of these are children, the elderly, and African Americans. But this statistic occurs in a society that in the last decade has witnessed unparalleled growth in the wealth of services, information, and consumer choices, especially in the realm of health. One just has to think of the number of pharmacies that have sprung up in your neighborhood, whether it's in a large city or small town. One would suppose that our health is being properly serviced. So why are we losing the battle for people's general well-being as is shown by recent data?

Looking back, the United States experienced many depressing events in the past century: the Depression, two world wars, and many smaller wars that directly affected the well-being and mental health of its citizenry. But somehow they were able to cope without being labeled "ill." They may have experienced many painful moments, but these didn't require medications or therapies, in general. Today, in a time of unprecedented prosperity, however, more and more people are being classified as incapable with coping with their daily routines and circumstances, and therefore, require treatment, usually in the form of pharmaceuticals.

Now into this contemporary situation is dropped an informational bomb. In 2008, the *New England Journal of Medicine* announced that recent studies show that placebos (sugar pills) can often be just as effective at improving mood, and even brain chemistry, as some of the most widely advertised and prescribed drugs in the country. This story echoes other similar studies, where other scientists disproved the effectiveness of Prozac and Zoloft in 1997 and 2002. Now many psychological critics are asking why do we continue to prescribe antidepressants when we've known for a decade that they don't work?

These reports stressed that placebos have been underestimated as a form of treatment for depression. But we think the more relevant insight gleaned from these results is that the patients aren't really sick, ill, or "depressed" in the first place. These studies, if interpreted in this light, then reveal a very disturbing pattern: we are pathologizing life. In this chapter we will show, by examining trends in medication for children, African Americans, and the elderly, that our claim is not hysterical, but it is the professional functionaries on sociology, psychology, psychiatry, and medicine that can be accused of overreacting and consequently overprescribing for normal moods, feelings, and sensations—in other words, the average spectrum of reactions to being alive.

For example, as we navigate our way into the 21st century, there is an ominous trend that, strangely, doesn't seem to concern people as much as it should: millions of children are now taking psychotropic drugs. And they're not doing it illegally but by prescription. In fact, the medical and educational establishments are conducting a skyrocketing campaign to get kids, and their parents, to "just say yes" to brain-altering pharmaceuticals, with the drug of choice being Ritalin. In 1970, when approximately 150,000 students were on Ritalin, America was alarmed enough to get the Drug Enforcement Agency to classify Ritalin and other amphetamine-type drugs as Class II substances, a category that includes cocaine and one that indicates a significant risk of abuse. Despite this apparent safeguard, the number of children taking psychiatric stimulants today has risen over fortyfold; current estimates are that between six and seven million children are taking them. The American Academy of Pediatrics estimates that as many as 3.8 million children, mostly boys, are currently diagnosed with attention hyperactivity disorder, and that at least a million children take Ritalin, a figure that many regard as a gross underestimate. And it is not just schoolchildren who are being dosed with psychotropics: even preschoolers, those aged two to four, experienced a tripling of such prescriptions in a recent five-year period.

Exactly why is all this juvenile pill-popping a problem? Well, for one thing, Ritalin is a drug that has a more powerful effect on the brain than cocaine. And we're supposed to be a country that eschews the use of such mind-altering substances, especially for children. For another, Ritalin's side effects can range from unwelcome personality changes to cardiovascular problems and death. Plus there's the very real issue of whether the "diseases" for which this powerful medicine is prescribed are in fact diseases at all.

The problem becomes further complicated when you consider that, in addition to the Ritalin explosion, increasing numbers of children are also being prescribed antidepressants, and that these are drugs originally designed and tested for adults. (A fact not generally publicized is that it's legal to prescribe drugs "off label," that is, for conditions or populations that they weren't originally designed for.) So in 1996, over 700,000 children and adolescents were taking Prozac and similar antidepressants in the SSRI group, an 80 percent increase from just two years earlier. It's not that the SSRIs have been proven effective in battling childhood and adolescent depression. They haven't. Nevertheless, today, the number of prescriptions has surpassed one million.

NO MORE DEPRESSION OR ANXIETY

Psychiatrist Peter Breggin estimates that each year, 10 percent of the school age population will take one or more psychiatric drugs. Some children are prescribed with several at once. And the phenomenon continues to grow, despite having disturbing evidence of severe induced personality changes, manic reactions, and psychotic behavior.

Medication advocates would argue that those children who are prescribed psychotropic drugs do in fact need them. Children with affective disturbances or attention deficits can focus better, and thus, learn better when medicated, they say. Opponents protest that the efficacy and safety of these drugs have not been proven, and some, further, believe that many psychiatric "conditions" exist only as labels in the minds of psychologists. Whether or not these conditions are real, one must agree that the exceedingly high numbers of prescriptions written for children in recent years are a cause for grave concern. And they're of concern not just to the children and parents directly touched by individual diagnoses, but to society at large. Consider the Columbine massacre and the rash of other school shootings that have rocked this country recently. As the *Washington Times Insight Magazine* reports, "the common link in the high school shootings may be psychotropic drugs like Ritalin and Prozac." For example, in 1998, 14-year-old Kip Kinkle killed his parents and then went on a shooting spree at his Springfield, Oregon high school, killing 2 and injuring 22. He was being treated with Ritalin and Prozac. Then there was the 15-year-old taking Ritalin who in 1999 wounded six classmates at Heritage High School in Georgia, and the 18-year-old who raped and murdered a 7-year-old girl in 1997, one week after starting to take Dexadrine. Even more recently, there's the case of Christopher Pitt, who, after switching onto Zoloft, murdered his own grandparents following the instructions of voices. One can't help but ask whether psychotropic drugs are dangerous not just to those taking them, but also, in some cases, to "innocent bystanders."

And there are some other basic questions people are beginning to ask as well: Do all these sick children need to be taking all these drugs? Are they really sick?

By far, the overwhelming majority of psychotropic prescriptions for children are given for attention deficit disorder (ADD) or attention hyperactivity disorder (ADHD). In some instances, taking medicine is a prerequisite for attending school, with refusal to comply considered grounds for dismissal, or worse, removal of the child from the home by the state. This outrages Fred Baughman, a board-certified child neurologist trained at New York University and Mount Sinai, and a fellow of the American Academy of Neurology. Baughman feels that it's one thing for a court to intervene and take over as legal guardian in a case where a child's life is truly at risk, but quite another thing when psychotropic drugs are forced upon children who don't fit into the mold. For instance, Baughman says, for religious reasons parents may refuse a needed blood transfusion for a child, or they may refuse to allow treatment for diabetes—a real disease—with insulin, a real treatment. The courts may have to intervene in such cases. But courts should have no place in mandating that behavioral problems in children be treated with drugs. "There are no physical or chemical abnormalities in these children," Baughman states. "The idea that there is a false belief spouted by psychiatry... For courts to intervene and to mandate such medical emergencies, is leading to tyranny over parents of normal children... When we're talking about... so-called psychiatric disorders, none of them are actual diseases due to physical abnormalities within the child," states Baughman.

An important argument against the thesis that ADHD and ADD are actual conditions is that the epidemic appears to be confined to North America. The use of Ritalin and similar prescriptions is overwhelmingly concentrated in the United

States and Canada. In fact, these two countries account for 96 percent of their use throughout the world, and children in the U.S. have been estimated to be from 10 to 50 times more likely to be labeled as having ADD than their counterparts in Britain or France. In American public schools, about 10 percent of all children in grades K–12 carries an ADHD diagnosis. Europe, by contrast, has a fraction of 1 percent so labeled. Could the United States and Canada really be so unique in the recent drastic upsurge of this malady?

Many in the health field are calling for more research in this area. For instance, Tomas Moore, senior fellow in health policy at George Washington University Medical Center, who feels that brain damage from Ritalin is more common than has been reported, often questions the rationale of giving Ritalin to children, stating that the chemical imbalance theory has not been established by scientific evidence. And while the public is given information by the National Institutes of Mental Health that ADHD is neurobiological in nature, NIMH psychiatrist Peter Jensen stated in 1996, "The National Institutes of Mental Health does not have an official position on whether ADHD is a neurobiological disorder." In other words, this agency is talking out of both sides of their mouth—not that this is an uncommon phenomenon in Washington.

Psychologist Diane McGuiness summed up the situation in 1991 by saying, "We have invented a disease, given it a medical sanction, and now we must disown it. The major question is: how do we go about destroying the monster we created? It is not easy to do this and still save face."

Psychologist Daniel Elkind in his 1981 classic, *The Hurried Child*, discussed the increasing "industrialization" of our schools with their regimented schedules, even at the elementary level, and their focus on turning out quality-controlled products, i.e., students. Today, with administrators under the gun to have their students perform well on standardized tests, and with more troubled children in the schools, the atmosphere has not gotten more relaxed. The inescapable fact is that schools have an interest in keeping order and children quiet and calm so that they can get on with the business of teaching and learning. And the psychiatric medicines do help keep schoolchildren under control. In the words of developmental pediatrician Dr. Joseph Keeley, "We sometimes use medications to make kids fit into schools rather than schools to fit the kids." Of course, there are better ways to make schools work such as appropriate therapy for troubled youngsters, custom-tailored education plans, and small classes. But these approaches are more difficult, and more expensive. Thus, the school district may have a vested interest in medication as a quick, less costly fix, although this may not be the best for a particular child. Says Dr. David Stein, "The drugs blunt their behavior. They don't act out in class, and they sit there quietly... The difficulty is that children learn nothing from the drug."

Schools justify the need for medications by saying that the children on Ritalin learn better because the drug allows them to focus, but that claim has never been proven. According to Stein, so-called ADD children can never learn when they want to; it's just that schools expect too much from students and do not engage them. "This country has started teaching second and third grade material in kindergarten, and children begin to get burnt out by the time they're in the second grade. They wind up hating schoolwork. And that's the key. These children can play very complex video games, they can read the instructions, because they enjoy doing it."

The situation in American schools was chillingly illustrated by a teacher with whom I talked recently. She works for a state-funded organization that sends teachers, social workers, and psychologists to disadvantaged schools for support. Once a week, she explained, there are meetings with the principal, other staff, and sometimes parents to discuss specific problem children. "Although we are given no specific training in how to advise or function as a team," she said, "we are looked at as experts, and our advice is highly regarded. In my experience, the meetings are merely attempts to find quick-fix solutions, and since the psychologist dominates, the answer to a great many childhood problems is an ADHD or ADD diagnosis for which medication is considered the logical solution."

This teacher told me she would never forget an experience she had when she was fairly new to team meetings:

> After another teacher had expressed concern about an active second grader, the psychologist and psychology intern reported findings to the parents at a team meeting. They said that the boy fit the ADHD class and couldn't sit still without fidgeting. They suggested that he should be taken to the doctor for a follow-up.
>
> The mother initially asked an intelligent question: "Will the doctor perform a special kind of test to determine that my son has a medical disorder?" The team could not answer that question in the affirmative since no such test is performed. The doctor merely observes the child's behavior, looks at the behavior checklist filled out by the parent and teacher, and then fills out the prescription.
>
> While the mother appeared immediately receptive to persuasion, the quiet father wore an expression of concern in his eyes. The principal asked what was wrong, and the father responded in one word: "Ritalin." The team then turned their attention to soothing the father, saying that medication would be in the boy's best interest because once he was calm he would be able to pay attention to

his schoolwork and succeed in his studies.

When the meeting ended, the teacher said, she pulled the father aside and told him she understood his concerns. "I told him that many parents were opposed to medicating their children and that alternative approaches did exist. Then I handed him a brochure on alternative approaches." She felt that she had to take a discreet approach because she'd learned from past meetings that it was useless to speak up. The psychologists are so married to their ideology that they're quick to shoot down the opposition. "Even though I attempted to be confidential," she reported, "the room was small, and I could feel the psychologist's eyes glaring at me, as if she was going to use the information to report me to the thought-control police."

Once the parents left, the teacher went on to relate, the red-faced principal exclaimed, "That burns me up! Here we are trying so hard to help their son, and the father gives us a hard time." Obviously, the principal did not understand why the idea of medicating a young child, possibly every day for the rest of his life, should concern parents.

Soon after that, the parents complied. The next time this teacher saw the second-grader in her math group, he was already on Ritalin, so she was able to see a before-and-after contrast in personality. The child had been a bit antsy before, calling out or even getting out of his seat from time to time, but his behavior seemed normal. Now the child seemed severely depressed. He would cry from the smallest slight, losing a turn in a board game, for example, and even crawl under the table to cry. He had never acted that way before. On one occasion, he told the teacher he wanted to kill himself. She reported that to the psychologist, who seemed annoyed at the trouble. Soon the psychologist reported back to the teacher that the parents didn't notice any difference in behavior. He would continue as before.

This teacher went on to make the point that biological "treatments" for childhood social disorders are not discriminatory—she has seen the same arrogance and insensitivity in an affluent school district on the other side of town. In the high school where she worked as a reading specialist, teachers confronted with children they deem problematic routinely say to peers and parents, "He [or she] should be on meds." The students' perceived problems can range from inability to focus to acting out to just not being able to read. Some parents do seem aware of the ADD controversy, but overall there is a blind acceptance of ADD as a true medical condition that requires medication.

It should be noted that it's not just elementary and high schools that seem to need a drug to help them run smoothly, but preschools and day care centers also. As writer Robyn Suriano recently pointed out in the *Orlando Sentinel*, the drug [Ritalin] reached its heyday in the 1990s, after more children started attending day care. "In a preschool, kids must follow instructions and behave just like older children in classrooms. Rambunctious ones are not easily tolerated in these surroundings, where workers must watch many children." This is not to say that day care centers are necessarily bad, but there are a lot of inadequately staffed and poorly equipped ones. These trap preschoolers in confining, boring situations for 10 hours a day and then complain when they act like the active, inquisitive, and needy young creatures that children just barely out of babyhood normally are. That drugs are used to remedy this situation is unconscionable, especially considering that Ritalin's label warns that the drug is only for those aged six and over. But an "off-label" prescription is legal, and it's happening. As a *Wall Street Journal* article reported, the use of prescription drugs to control toddlers' behavior has increased dramatically in the past decade.

The *Journal* article did give voice to a couple of dissenting professionals concerning this trend. Psychiatrist Joseph Coyle, chairman of the Department of Psychiatry at Harvard Medical School, was one. The brains of young children are developing rapidly, he pointed out, and the drugs can alter the process. Coyle also cited the financial interests of managed care in creating a system in which doctors are too busy to do much more than prescribe. And Dr. Julie Zito, an associate professor at the University of Maryland's School of Pharmacy, was especially skeptical of the use of Ritalin in two-year-olds. "What is abnormally inattentive in a two-year-old?" she asked.

It was Dr. Zito who, along with colleagues from the University of Maryland, Johns Hopkins, and Kaiser Permanente's Center for Health Research, authored a study on "Trends in the Prescribing of Psychotropic Medications to Preschoolers." Published in the *Journal of the American Medical Association,* the study contained some unsettling findings concerning very young children and psychotropic drugs. The researchers found that poor—and particularly black—children are being prescribed Ritalin at a younger and younger age. A 300 percent increase on prescriptions to the very young between 1991 and 1995 was cited. The study also mentioned Prozac is being given to children younger than one year of age to the tune of 3,000 prescriptions in 1994.

Before ADD and ADHD came into vogue, amphetamines were seldom prescribed. Ritalin was given for narcolepsy, a rare neurological disorder that causes people to fall asleep unexpectedly despite adequate sleep, but sales were miniscule. Now, thanks to the popularity of ADD and ADHD, Ritalin sales are significantly healthier. Moreover, the psychiatric establishment has seemingly discovered several other childhood disorders, including pediatric depression, for which medications are routinely prescribed. By the way, most of the people prescribing psychiatric drugs are not psychiatrists, but primary care physicians, who have not received the kind of sophisticated mental health training needed to understand what's involved in prescribing these life-altering substances. Our managed care system of health care bears at least some of the blame for this trend. In 2001, an article called "Generation Rx" appeared in *Parents* magazine. It pointed out, "Here, as with almost everything else in the tangled world of health care, economics plays a decisive role. Drugs have become the treatment of first resort when kids exhibit behavioral problems, partly because most managed-care plans readily cover the cost of medication but often won't pay for long-term alternative treatments such as talk or behavioral therapy."

Some of the people who manage managed care are not particularly interested in getting to the source of patient's problems, focused as they are on the bottom line and the quick fix. Psychiatrist Dr. David Kaiser elaborates, "When I talk to a managed health care representative about the care of one of my patients, they invariably want to know about medications I am using and little else, and there is often an implication that I am not medicating aggressively enough. There is now a growing cottage industry within psychiatry in advocating ways to work with managed care, despite the obvious fact that managed care has little interest in quality care and realistic approaches to real patients. This financial pressure by managed care contributes added pressure for psychiatry to go down a biological road and to avoid more realistic treatment approaches."

The boom in psychiatric drug sales has been helped along by a vigorous marketing campaign. Psychiatrist Loren Mosher reports that at meetings of the American Psychiatric Association, drug companies "basically lease 90 percent of the exhibition space and spend huge sums in giveaway items. They have nearly completely squeezed out the little guys, and the symposiums that once were dedicated to scientific reports now have been replaced by the pharmaceutical-industry-sponsored speakers." And pitches for drugs are made not just to medical practitioners, but also to teachers and parents. In the early 1990s, pharmaceutical companies distributed pamphlets to schools nationwide on how to diagnose ADHD and ADD, conditions for which medication was presented as the solution. During this time, America saw a dramatic rise in Ritalin consumption, close to a 700 percent increase. Ritalin's manufacturer also funded CHADD to encourage parents to support the drug solution and to keep public confidence levels high. Today, drug companies continue to spend hundreds of thousands of dollars on ads in psychiatric journals.

They've also started advertising in popular magazines. Recently, some stimulant manufacturers have gone against standard international practice and begun marketing directly to parents. Here's how a 2001 *New York Times* article called "Schools' Backing of Behavior Drugs Comes Under Fire" describes this appalling trend:

> In the back-to-school section of this month's *Ladies' Home Journal,* tucked among the ads for Life cereal, bologna and Jell-O pudding, are three full-page advertisements for the A.D.H.D. treatments. The ads evoke a sense of Rockwellian calm. Children chat happily next to a school bus. A child's hand gently touches the hand of an adult. In one, for the new drug Metadate CD, an approving mother embraces her beaming son as the drug itself is named and promoted.
>
> This is a first. Metadate CD, like Ritalin, Adderall and similar drugs, are what are known as Schedule II controlled substances, the most addictive substances that are still legal. (Schedule I drugs like heroin and LSD are illegal.) In keeping with a 1971 international treaty, such controlled

substances have never been marketed directly to consumers, only to doctors. There is, however, no federal law to prevent drug companies from doing it. Yet the new magazine advertisement by Celltech Pharmaceuticals, the British maker of Metadate CD, states, "Introducing Metadate capsules. One dose covers his A.D.H.D for the whole school day."

According to *The Times*, in the year 2000 close to 20 million prescriptions were written for ADD medicines, with sales bringing in about $758 million. The rise in ADD diagnoses has been most dramatic among our youth. In the last 10 years, prescriptions to treat ADD in 10- to 19-year-olds rose 86 percent, which mean 7.8 million teens are being drugged unnecessarily. It is true that a lot of this profit goes into research that tests the drugs' safety and efficacy. The obvious down side to this, though, is that with companies funding their own testing, the results can be biased, as it is not in the company's best interest to get negative results that discourage business.

This conflict-of-interest situation raises ethical issues that are especially troublesome when you consider that children are the targets of these drug companies. Furthermore, today it's not just the classic "problem child" who is being targeted for stimulant consumption. As Peter Breggin points out in *Talking Back to Ritalin*, there is a wide range of children being given stimulants, from the truly hyperactive child with severe behavioral problems to a child who is simply dreamy or inattentive. As is the case with other psychotropics, the net of this drug's reach seems to have widened.

Many children taking Ritalin will develop involuntary muscle contractions and limb movements known as tics, or dyskinesia. A study published in the *Archives of Pediatric and Adolescent Medicine* showed that this can happen to up to 9 percent of children taking stimulants. Other studies in the peer-reviewed medical literature bear out this association, as well as the Ritalin-psychosis connection. Ritalin has also been shown to have an adverse effect on heart tissue and has been linked to cancer. In the mid-'90s, the FDA forced Ritalin's maker to send letters to 100,000 doctors, warning them of a possible link between drug and liver cancer. Researchers reported to the FDA that their studies show "clear evidence" that link the drug to cancer. The FDA changed the warning to "some evidence," a change that was protested by one of the main researchers. A formal proposal to keep the wording "clear evidence" was presented to an FDA panel, but this was defeated by a vote of four to three. "Clear evidence" became "some evidence," and ultimately the FDA publicly announced that there was a "weak link" between Ritalin and cancer and that doctors should not be concerned about continuing to prescribe the drug.

A problem that some children and teenagers experience with Ritalin is called "rebound." When the drug is metabolized and the level in the bloodstream goes down, these children seem to go back to a hyperactive state "and then some." They may get excitable or impulsive, or develop insomnia. In fact, as many as half the so-called ADHD children on medication reported some presleep agitation. Physicians try to handle this problem by decreasing the last dose of the day, or, alternatively, adding another dose, so that the child sleeps with a new supply of Ritalin in his blood. Sometimes this works, but one has to wonder about the advisability of children taking a sleep-pattern-altering drug over the long term. Yet another Ritalin side effect is the stunting of growth, which occurs in some children taking moderate to high stimulant dosages over a period of years. This happens not just because stimulants can diminish appetite, but also because they may alter the body's natural balance of growth hormones. The growth-stunting phenomenon doesn't seem to have alarmed the medical establishment as much as it should. Consider the advice given by clinical psychologist Dr. John Taylor in his book *Helping Your Hyperactive/Attention Deficit Child*. The author notes, first, that some physicians recommend taking the child off of medication during vacation periods, so that he can catch up in height and weight. Then Taylor counsels: "The crucial question is whether your child's behavior can be tolerated if he or she is unmedicated (or undermedicated) during the summer months. Several adjustments are available. Your child can play outdoors more, attend camps, participate in athletic programs or other vigorous play activities, or even be sent to live with a relative. There is little or no requirement for intense academic pursuit, there is no need to sit still for hours as is required in school, and summer entertainments can take advantage of your child's interests to prevent boredom... Among those who are not given any medication-free periods and who experience the stunting effect, the average amount is less than two inches. If stunting occurs and becomes an important psychological issue, choice of hair style and footwear can compensate."

At least three questions arise. First, if it's possible to give a child a stimulating and active life in the summer, at camp, or with relatives, why can't this be done in the winter, in school, and with a nuclear family? Surely arranging for more outdoor playtime and more interesting activities is preferable to putting a child on drugs. Second, do parents and doctors have the right to stunt a child's growth for any other reason than, perhaps, to save his life? And third, even if "choice of hairstyle and footwear can compensate," for decreased height, how is the child going to feel about this later, when he finds out what's been done to him?

In addition to all the potentially damaging effects of Ritalin, one has to factor in the reality that it doesn't work. Yes, it does make some children better behaved at certain times. But there are no studies showing improved academic performance or social behavior over the long term. What *has* been shown is that the side effects can be quite serious.

Most people assume that medications are proven safe before they are marketed. But this is not always the case, especially when you consider the long-term picture. Science knows very little about the long-term effects of medicating children. In effect, children have become guinea pigs. The results of this grand experiment are only now becoming evident, and sometimes the consequences can be deadly. Consider the case of Stephanie Hall, a first grader placed on Ritalin because her teacher felt she was "just a little bit too antsy," according to her mother. "The teacher suggested that Stephanie go for testing, so we went the route of a neurologist who said she could throw a ball and read a book and psychologist who said she had average intelligence but, yes, she was a little easily distracted. So now she qualifies to be medicated." When she turned 12, the prescription was increased; that very day, Stephanie died from cardiac arrest in her sleep. Says her mom, "Her death was caused by cardiac arrhythmia with no family history of any type of heart problem whatsoever, and she died a day after her medication had been increased. It kind of adds up."

A double tragedy struck the Hall family when Stephanie's sister, Jenny, also a longtime Ritalin user, started to have seizures. Subsequent medical tests revealed a brain tumor. Mrs. Hall believes Jenny was misdiagnosed; as a result proper medical attention was delayed. She states, "There's Jenny's ADHD; it's a brain tumor... But there's a chance that the child could have an underlying neurological disease that really needs treatment." Mrs. Hall also wonders whether the medication could have precipitated or exacerbated Jenny's condition: "It probably made her condition worse because prior to being on medication, she never had seizures. I later read that if you have a low threshold to seizures, you should never take Ritalin to begin with." She and her husband are now suing Novartis, the maker of Ritalin, for producing a defective product, and concealing adverse reactions and deaths related to its use.

In a more publicized story, Matthew Smith, a 14-year-old from Michigan, had also, like Stephanie Hall, been taking Ritalin from the time he was in first grade. After eight years of ingesting the drug daily, Matthew suddenly became pulseless and died while riding his scooter. An autopsy performed by the county medical examiner, a Dr. Dragovic, found that Matthew's heart muscle was diffusely replaced with scar tissue, as were the muscular walls of the coronary vessels. Much to the displeasure of the psychiatric and pharmaceutical industry, the doctor publically stated Matthew's death was undoubtedly due to the heart damage akin to that regularly seen in deaths among amphetamine addicts, and that his death was clearly due to Ritalin.

Yet another incident occurred in a psychiatric facility near San Antonio, Texas, where young Randy Steel was being restrained when he suddenly died. Randy was on several psychiatric drugs at the time. But his first psychiatric diagnosis, his entry into a life of psychiatry, had been ADHD, and his first drug was Dexedrine or dextroamphetamine. At the time of death, he had an enlarged heart.

It should surprise no one to learn that Ritalin and other amphetamines can lead to death. The dangers are well known to doctors who study the adverse effects of these substances as medical students. Dr. Dragovic explains: "Methylphenidate—that's Ritalin's chemical name—is classified as an adrenergic agonist. This is a type of drug that boosts the adrenergic system. It affects everything that has as its chemical pathway adrenalin, noradrenaline, dopamine, those types of mediators and transmitters. Drugs in the category of stimulants also include Ritalin's cousins—amphetamines, methamphetamines, and even cocaine. If they are repetitively used, the drugs stimulate the adrenergic system in the human body. Over a period of time...many months to many years, the enhancement of the adregenic system will produce changes in small blood vessels. Some cells will be lost, and in an attempt to repair the area there will be scarring... The blood vessels will narrow. The changes that we're seeing in kids who have been on Ritalin for about eight years are basically the same as changes in someone that has been abusing cocaine regularly over a period of years."

Dragovic adds that irreversible damage to the vascular system could also result in cardiovascular problems down the road, including high blood pressure. By medicating vast numbers of children today, we could be creating an army of future patients with other conditions that need to be treated. "Do we need that?" asks Dr. Dragovic. His answer is certainly no, but as he explains, "that's the peril of chronic Ritalin use, or of any stimulant for that matter. It's paying the dues in long-term use."

There are few if any statistics on how many people experience adverse effects. What we do know is that, according to the FDA adverse reaction reports, which are notoriously incomplete, there were 160 Ritalin-related deaths between 1990 and 1997, most of them cardiovascular related. We know that Ritalin is a vasoactive (blood-vessel-altering) substance that decreases cerebral blood flow. And we know that children's brains are undergoing dramatic development through the teen years, not just in early childhood, as had been previously thought. We also know that Ritalin can have persistent, cumulative effects on the myocardium, the muscle cells that form most of the heart wall. With all these facts in mind, one has to wonder the implications for the millions of American children being dosed over the long term with stimulants. As Dr. Fred Baughman points out, "There is no way of knowing the actual frequency of...any medical side effects of these drugs, because there is no required reporting system. There is only a voluntary system whereby physicians would call the FDA, and needless to say, they don't often report their own implications." Ritalin's fast growth—it's legal and illegal use—could mean that a multitude of tragedies are on the horizon.

There are those who believe that what we perceive as ADHD in many young children and teenagers is simply our youth's natural reaction to the sped-up quality to much of American life today. One of these people is psychologist Dr. Richard DeGrandpre, fellow of the National Institute on Drug Abuse and author of *Ritalin Nation*: "As society goes faster, so do the rhythms of our own consciousness. This is especially true for children, who grow up in concert with the latest speed."

DeGrandpre points out that young people who have known nothing but a hurried, perpetually wired environment, will tend to get restless when the stimulation level lags—in a classroom, for instance. And he says that Ritalin, being itself a stimulant, does not so much erase the need for excitement but rather fulfill it, in a prosthetic way. Indeed, he coins the phrase "prosthetic pharmacology" to refer the way modern psychiatry uses drugs as crutches rather than cures. And while a real crutch may help an injured person's leg heal, psychiatric crutches often mask underlying problems, resulting in no effort to deal with them.

A noteworthy point made by DeGrandpre is that, while years ago, the condition then known as hyperactivity tended to disappear when childhood ended, today's ADHD seems to linger into adolescence and adulthood for a lot of its "victims." But why would a bona fide disorder suddenly affect a whole new age group? There has to be a cultural component in play.

We don't seem to want to face any cultural concerns, though. We'd rather diagnose a large segment of the population as mentally impaired, thereby shifting our mental well-being away from society and toward the medical profession. When people are identified as "sick," their issues are seen as the result of a diseased mind, rather than as a reaction to an unhealthy family dynamic or social environment. But one need only compare the world today to that of 50 years ago to appreciate the magnitude of the additional stresses in contemporary times that could result in maladaptive behavior. Many children practically grow up in day-care centers, for example, their parents being too busy or hassled to raise them, and dinner is usually eaten in front of the TV. Family members don't interact with each other. School demands more academic work from children at an earlier age. The extended family is practically nonexistent, with grandparents, aunts, and uncles living many states away. As a result, values are not taught to children. The divorce rate is approaching 67 percent, and 50 percent of children are being raised by single parents. These statements about modern life are almost cliché, but the fact remains that the environment they describe does have an impact on children.

I believe you have to look deeply at the values of society to really understand what ails its people. In today's America, it seldom occurs to anyone that it's okay to just be by being. In our society we hate the idea of being without purpose. Baby boomers, in particular, feel that we're always supposed to have a purpose, a goal, a motivation to get there, discipline to keep the motivation going, and passion to fuel it all. We're supposed to value success and competition. But in the process of doing all that we frequently lose our sense of identity. We have to consider that when today's kids take a careful look at their parents, they may not want to duplicate what they see. They—or at least some of them—may be turned off by the high-stress levels, the judgmental attitudes, the lack of quality of life, the lack of unconditional love, the absence of peace of mind, and the inability to feel comfortable with what is. So kids may say, "I'm just going to kind of hang out in the moment." And we think, "No you can't, you've got to get in there. You've got to achieve. You've got to prove yourself. You're up against competition. There's a shortage of everything." And then we put them in a situation where they can't win and can only be labeled as having some sort of deficit.

An alien observer looking at the current drug situation in the United States would certainly be confused. On the one hand, we're preaching drug avoidance to our youth. On the other, we're dosing a lot of them with mind-altering drugs, which as we've just seen, can sometimes tragically alter behavior as well.

One of the results of our eagerness to fix problems with drugs is the widespread abuse of drugs that have been legally prescribed to children. According to the DEA, Ritalin and other stimulants are among the most frequently stolen prescription medicines, with pills often crushed and snorted for an immediate high. Ritalin is now a prime choice among the drugs abused on college campuses across the country. High school students use it recreationally as well. A 1997 Indiana University survey reported that nearly 7 percent of high school students had engaged in this practice.

It's time to reassess what we want for our children. Do we want to bring them up in a drug culture or not? Do we want to mold them in the confines of our educational system, or do we want to fashion an education that will respond to *their* needs? What are our criteria for a successful child? And will we continue to label those who don't meet these criteria as psychologically abnormal? We're sticking this label onto an awful lot of kids lately.

An important point was made in *Contemporary Directions in Psychopathology*, a textbook used to train psychiatrists. It was stated that there was "evidence that the current psychiatric diagnosis system is a reflection of social, cultural developments rather than scientific data." The editor of this book, Gerald Clerman, also edited *The Archives of General Psychiatry* and sat on the American Psychiatric Association's task force for its *Diagnostic and Statistical Manual of Mental Disorders*—the "psychiatrist's bible" of diagnostic labels. So basically, in a totally "establishment" textbook, we have an admission that social and cultural expectations, rather than objective science, form the basis for the way we evaluate who is mentally abnormal.

We would do well to remember this—and then rethink our penchant for labeling—before we prescribe any more brain altering drugs to children.

In light of our theme that the mental health industry is pathologizing life—a very broad category—then we would have to look at the other side of the spectrum, the elderly, to see if our argument applies.

> A woman in her 70s copes with recurring bouts of depression after the death of her beloved husband. She consults a psychiatrist who tells her all she needs to bring her out of the dark is ECT, electroconvulsive therapy. What he fails to consider is that the patient has a weak heart, and the consent form she signs mentions nothing of the risk. The woman allows herself to undergo treatment and, days later, dies.

This particular scenario is made up, but variations on it happen all too frequently. Consider that half the 100,000 Americans being shocked each year are senior citizens. Now consider records from Texas, the only state required to track complications within two weeks of ECT administration. These records document a death rate of ECT of 1 in 200 recipients of the treatment. Statistics also reveal that the typical candidate for ECT is a depressed middle- or upper-middle-class woman in her 70s who checks herself into a private hospital. The targeted population has shifted since the 1950s and '60s, when schizophrenic men in their 40s were the primary group subjected to ECT, and the reason was economics. Insurance no longer supports long hospital stays, but Medicare, the government's medical insurance for people 65 and older, will generously reimburse psychiatrists who administer ECT. This incentive is apparent once again in Texas records, which show 65-year-olds receiving 360 percent more shock therapy than 64-year-olds.

But paralleling the growth of ECT is the growing number of critics of the treatment, both within and outside the psychiatric establishment. Shock is not just ineffective, the opposition claims, it often leaves recipients in a worsened condition than before treatment. Depression and suicidal ideation soon return, complicated by ECT-induced brain damage and memory loss. Plus new conditions, such as epilepsy and heart arrhythmias, can develop. Moreover, signing the permission form for this treatment may be signing your life away, as the risk of death during or soon after the procedure is great, far higher than ECT proponents admit, in part due to the targeting of fragile elderly populations. ECT's most ardent challengers, often former patients themselves, wonder how healing professionals could have forgotten their Hippocratic oath to do no harm. They assert that ECT is a barbaric procedure that must be banned.

But why has ECT had a revival? Consider that sixty years ago, once ECT was adopted in the U.S., abuse of this modality became common. This is not to say that the treatment is not in and of itself an abuse, but from the 1940s to the '70s, shock treatments were often given in psychiatric hospitals not just as treatment, but to quiet or punish patients. In 1996 *Washington Post* article called "Shock Therapy...It's Back" one woman remarked of her experience in the early 1970s: "I wasn't depressed; I wasn't suicidal... They were shocking everyone on the ward—the young, the really old, everyone... What were they shocking us for? Ward control? Medical historian David J. Rothman of Columbia University points out that ECT stands practically alone among medical/surgical interventions in its role as a patient control mechanism used for the benefit of the hospital staff."

Economic factors of the 1980s brought ECT into the limelight once again, particularly insurance policies that refused to pay for lengthy procedures like ECT. Since then, electroshock has received glowing endorsements from numerous organizations, including the National Institutes for Health, the National Alliance for the Mentally Ill, the National Depressive and Manic Depressive Association, and the American Psychological Association. This last organization takes an active role in ECT advocacy. This includes fighting attempts to restrict the procedure and working to relax current standards so that shock therapy will become an initial, rather than last-resort, treatment for the depressed.

Although present-day modifications can help in certain ways by reducing a patient's fear and stopping flailing movements that can cause bone fractures, the treatment itself—the zapping of the brain with an electrical current—is the same as it had been and inevitably results in brain damage. According to the National Head Injury Foundation, each treatment equals one moderate-to-severe head injury. And as a series of shocks are prescribed—eight to fifteen on average and as many as one per month on an indefinite basis—the wounding intensifies. In 1983, Dr. Sydney Samant described what happens in the following way: "As a neurologist and an electroencephalographer, I have seen many patients after ECT, and I have no doubt that ECT produces effects identical of those of a head injury. After multiple sessions of ECT, a patient has symptoms identical to those of a retired, punch-drunk boxer... After a few sessions of ECT, the symptoms are those of moderate cerebral contusion, and further enthusiastic use of ECT may result in the patient functioning at a subhuman level. Electroconvulsive therapy, in effect, may be defined as a controlled type of brain damage produced by electrical means."

The scientific literature is replete with research confirming memory damage from ECT as a rule rather than the exception. For example, in Freeman and Kendall's 1986 study, 74 patients mentioned "memory impairment" as a continuing problem, and "a striking 30 percent felt that their memory had been permanently affected." The authors mentioned that these symptoms were probably underreported because the patients were interviewed by the same doctor who treated them. An interesting note: the 1990 APA task force sites Freeman and Kendall—these same authors—as indicating "a small minority of patients, however, report persistent deficits." Once again, we see what is so common in today's proprietary science—those who run the studies also design the protocols and analyze the finished data. Those results should be set aside from those who analyze it later and may have a bias to overstate a statistic.

Cardiovascular complications arising out of ECT are commonly seen in the scientific literature. For instance, the *Journal of Clinical Psychiatry* reported that 28 percent of a group of 42 patients undergoing ECT suffered cardiovascular problems following treatment. Of the patients who already had a history or indication of cardiac disease, 70 percent developed cardiac complications. The *Journal of Humanistic Psychology* reported on a 57-year-old man who died of heart rupture after receiving several shock treatments." From the same article: "Physicians from Tulane University Medical School reported on a 69-year-old woman who developed brain hemorrhage during ECT. She was also left with epilepsy afterward. This was as expected, associated with further deterioration in her mental status from her baseline depression. They conclude that the fragile vessels of the elderly may make some patients a particularly high risk for ECT."

Psychiatrists hail electroshock as the best method for

curing affective disorders and preventing suicides. One of its most zealous proponents, Dr. Max Fink, a professor of psychiatry at the State University of New York at Stony Brook and the editor-in-chief of *Convulsive Therapy*, goes so far as to proclaim ECT as "God's gift to man," and has stated that "it should be given to all patients whose condition is severe enough to require hospitalization." A closer look, however, casts doubt on psychiatry's enthusiasm. To begin, one needs to ask what psychiatrists really mean when they call electroshock effective. For how long do patients show improvement from depression? What do the studies conclude about ECT and suicide prevention? And what do psychiatrists actually consider patient improvement?

What an ECT fact sheet fails to tell patients is that improvements are temporary. Studies have never concluded that patients remain depression-free for longer than a month. Initially ECT recipients score higher on the Hamilton depression scale, a test used to measure depression, but weeks later their scores drop again. This is why psychiatrists recommend follow-up treatments with antidepressants and more electroshock every few weeks. Maintenance with antidepressants does not guarantee success, according to one study published in the *New England Journal of Medicine*. The study reported a 59 percent return to depression two months following ECT.

Electroshock therapy is to psychiatrists what open-heart surgery and hysterectomy are to other branches of medicine—a lucrative income booster. Charges of several hundreds of dollars per treatment add up quickly, so that physicians shocking patients three times a week, for instance, can increase their salary by over $27,000 a year, and more ambitious doctors may receive a $200,000 bonus. With the electroshock industry grossing $2 to $3 billion a year, and psychiatric groups lobbying for relaxed restrictions, doctors have ample opportunity for financial gain.

Since most insurance policies permit month-long hospital

stays, a course of ECT may be begun right away. Or it may start a month later when major medical insurance kicks in for "major" treatment protocols, of which ECT is one. This second option is the best deal for private psychiatric facilities (where the bulk of ECT takes place), as beds remain filled longer for a charge of several thousand dollars per patient. Afterwards insurance will reimburse patients for outpatient follow-up procedures, in which people are drugged, shocked, wheeled into the recovery room while in a coma, and sent home in a stupor the very same day. The importance of insurance in influencing who gets treatment was noted by one psychiatrist, who stated, "Finding that the patient has insurance seemed like the most common indication for giving electroshock."

The fact is that anyone speaking to a psychiatrist is at risk of being perceived as psychopathological. All a psychiatrist needs to do is pick one or more conditions that seem to fit from the psychiatric "bible," the *DSM-IV*, where hundreds of so-called "diagnosable conditions" are listed—everything from insomnia, worry, caffeinism, to being shy. Very few of the "disorders" are organic; the majority are socially based.

In a rush to diagnose and treat, what psychiatry forgets is that mental symptoms can be caused by poor physical health. An example of misdiagnosis is the case of Ruth Reed Price, whose nervous breakdown resulted in the diagnosis of schizophrenia when the real problem, discovered later, was a thyroid imbalance. In her 1995 testimony on banning electroshock in Austin, Texas, Price talks of the damage to her memory and nervous system that made returning to work a nightmare. "Instead of trying to really discover what was wrong," she says, "the Austin State Hospital staff made a wrong assumption and proceeded to damage my brain and impair my memory with their violent electroshock therapy."

So, one of the effects of the new pathologizing of life itself today is that older technologies, even disgraced ones like

ECT, are retrieved as arsenal for this panicked invasion of our bodies. Another effect is that newer, alternative modalities, which acknowledge normal life experiences and emotions, are being avoided altogether.

• CHAPTER 4 •

Side Effects of Drugs

Most people do not question the advice of their physician and take whatever drugs are prescribed for them. Other doctors offer an alternative, but their patients, believing that medicine is their only recourse or unwilling to exert the effort necessary to change poor habits, will ask or even pressure their doctors for medication. Whatever the reason, our society is saturated with legal drug users, and this is causing us some grave problems.

Study after study reveals that properly prescribed medicines are having adverse effects. The statistics for how many people are injured, hospitalized, and even dying from their medications is staggering. Yet the numbers are understated because they reflect only the hospitals' reports of such incidents. What is not taken into account is the amount of people suffering from such incidents at home, where the vast majority of these drugs are taken. It has been estimated, in fact, that adverse incidences occur 28 times more at home than at hospitals.

In 2008, the Center for Disease Control and Prevention estimated that 26,000 people a year die from accidental prescription pill overdose. Apparently our paid medical professionals aren't skilled or interested enough to instruct their patients on how to properly and safely take the medications

Side Effects of Drugs

that they are so eager to prescribe. It is estimated that there are more than 100,000 deaths caused every year by the side effects of medication. You should reevaluate your personal health care physician to see how much they actually care about you as a patient.

To make matters worse, improperly prescribed medications are on the rise. Giving a two-year-old an antidepressant is medically unsound and unjustifiable. How in the world can you determine that a two-year-old is suffering from anxiety? You can't. The brain of a two-year-old is still developing, as is the brain of a three-, four-, five-, and six-year-old. Yet the greedy manufacturers of these drugs are targeting an ever-younger market.

Has anyone asked what studies have been done on brain development in children who have been taking these drugs for a period of years? The answer is none. Then how will you know what the consequences will be? The answer is no one does. What this means is the risk is borne purely by the patient, who can become a victim, and not by the physician or manufacturers.

In the current political light, it is not surprising that Eli Lilly was exempt from being sued for adding thimerosal mercury to vaccines under the Homeland Security Act of 2002. What in the world does suing a manufacturer for possible neurological effects from a vaccine additive have to do with homeland security? Nothing, but for the fact that Eli Lilly's CEO at the time, Sidney Taurel, also sat on the advisory board of the Homeland Security committee and had a strong political connection to George Bush Sr., who was on the board of Eli Lilly. The transactions are utterly transparent. But at the end of the day, we still have people receiving medications that should not be receiving them, and they are having adverse effects.

So whether you are taking a properly or improperly prescribed drug, the incidence of negative side effects numbers into the hundreds of thousands, and possibly into the millions. This means, quite simply, that the number one cause of death in the United States is not from heart disease and not from stroke, but from the medications that are prescribed by a physician.

We therefore need to give you some idea of how dangerous the various medical procedures and medications are. We go beyond just the psychiatric ones to show you that across the board, in virtually every specialization, there is an enormous amount of unproven and dangerous medical practice occurring. *Therefore caveat emptor, consumers beware.* This is not to suggest that all medications for any condition are inappropriate. Clearly, some are essential, and lifesaving. But compared to how many are offered it, is a relatively small number.

Beyond the pathologizing of life itself, the most devastating side effect of antidepressant drugs is perhaps the false hope that the antidepressants give. They will never cure the underlying cause of depression. Yet, people take them with some notion, some belief, some misguided hope—a false hope—that drugs will indeed solve all of their problems. Instead, these drugs cover up their symptoms and give people a false and synthetic sense of relief.

We also have to consider a whole generation of young people growing up on Ritalin who have had their behavior artificially modified from a very young age. They never learn how to deal with feelings of sadness, anger, joy, and accomplishment without the overlay of drugs. They have learned to equate drugs with how to cope and never learned how to be confident in their own abilities. As adults, they don't know how to deal with normal feelings. They get depressed and fall right into the trap of thinking they need something to help them feel better. Prozac or Zoloft or any one of the other Prozac sisters comes across loud and clear in sexy TV ads telling them they don't have to cope.

Beyond what Ritalin does to kids' moods, the *Journal of the American Medical Association* has remarked, "Ritalin acts much like cocaine."

According to the *New England Journal of Medicine*, since the mid-1990s, drug companies have tripled the amount of money they spend on advertising prescription drugs directly to consumers. The majority of the money is spent on dramatic television ads. From 1996 to 2000, spending rose from $791 million to nearly $2.5 billion. Authors of the *NEJM* paper admit that "there is no solid evidence on the appropriateness of prescribing that results from consumers requesting an advertised drug." The drug companies maintain that direct-to-consumer advertising is educational. But according to Dr. Sidney M. Wolfe of the Public Citizen Health Research Group in Washington, D.C., the public is often misinformed about these ads. It's inevitable that patients go to their doctors demanding to become the images they see on TV by asking for a drug when they really want to be like the actor they see on the screen. Doctors are placed in a terrible bind and some spend valuable clinic time trying to talk patients out of unnecessary drugs; others write the prescription. Dr. Wolfe points out in an editorial accompanying this paper that one study found that a "substantial proportion of people mistakenly believe that the FDA reviews all ads before they are released and allows only the safest and most effective drugs to be promoted directly to the public."

According to Sarah Boseley of the *Guardian*, "Scientist are accepting large sums of money from drug companies to put their names into articles endorsing new medicines that they have not written—a growing practice that some fear is putting scientific integrity in jeopardy." She continued, "Ghostwriting has become widespread in such areas of medicine as cardiology, and psychiatry, where drugs play a major role in treatment." In addition, Ms. Boseley interviewed Fuller Torrey, executive director of the Stanley Foundation

Research Program in Bethesda, Maryland. He found that British psychiatrists were being paid around $2,000 (£1,400) for each symposium talk, plus expenses, and Americans were paid between $3,000 and $10,000. Mr. Torrey is quoted as saying, "Some of us believe that the present system is approaching a high-class form of professional prostitution."

In 2000, Dr. Marcia Angell, former editor of the *New England Journal of Medicine,* wrote an article called "Is Academic Medicine for Sale?" She said that in one paper on antidepressants, the authors' financial ties to the manufacturers, which must be declared, were so extensive that she had to run them on the website. She said, "We found very few who did not have financial ties to drug companies that make antidepressants."

The World Health Organization's director of Essential Drugs and Medicines Policy, Jonathan Quick, wrote in a recent *WHO Bulletin*: "If clinical trials become a commercial venture in which self-interest overrules public interest and desire overrules science, then the social contract which allows research on human subjects in return for medical advances is broken."

In general, drugs are tested on individuals who are fairly healthy and not on other medications, which can interfere with findings. But when drugs are declared "safe" and let loose in society, they are going to be used by people on a lot of other medications with a lot of other health problems. Then science begins documenting the real effects. According to the General Accounting Office (an agency of the U.S. government), "GAO found that of the 198 drugs approved by the FDA between 1976 and 1985…102 (or 51.5 percent) had serious post-approval results…the serious post-approval risks [included] heart failure, myocardial infarction, anaphylaxis, respiratory depression and arrest, seizures, kidney and liver failure, severe blood disorders, birth defects and fetal toxicity, and blindness."

The History of Antidepressant Drugs and Their Side Effects

There are three main classes of antidepressant drugs: MAO inhibitors, tricyclic antidepressants, and selective serotonin reuptake inhibitors (SSRIs). The actions of all three rely on the fact that neurons depend on serotonin, a brain neurotransmitter, to convey messages through the nervous system. Research on serotonin has shown that some depressed people have low levels of serotonin in the brain. So, these drugs are given in order to enhance serotonin levels with the hope that this increase will alleviate depression. One of the main side effects of all the antidepressants is sexual dysfunction including impotence—both physically and psychologically. Patients don't want to have sex, and if they did want to, they can't.

MAO Inhibitors

MAO Inhibitors (monoamine oxidase inhibitors) were the first prescription antidepressants. They work by blocking an enzyme called monoamine oxidase, which acts to break down monoamines and eliminate them from the body. Powerful brain neurotransmitters like serotonin and norepinephrine are monoamines, and if you turn off the enzyme that breaks them down, the result is more molecules building up. The effect can be like taking an SSRI drug like Prozac. There are about a dozen MAO inhibitors, but the most common ones still used today are Parnate (tranylcypromine sulfate) and Nardil (phenelzine sulfate).

MAO inhibitors actually work more rapidly than the trycyclic antidepressants, but the side effects of MAO inhibitors have relegated them to the background of psychiatric drug intervention. MAO inhibitors interact with a chemical called tyramine, which must be broken down by monoamine oxidase enzymes. If you block the enzyme with an MAO inhibitor, then tyramine builds up. Tyramine causes elevation of blood pressure, which could lead to stroke and/or heart attack. And the major catch is that tyramine is found in a lot of common foods such as beer, legumes (e.g., fava and soy beans), fermented soy products, cheese, fish, ginseng, meat, sauerkraut, shrimp paste, soups, and yeast extracts.

Beyond high blood pressure, there is a long list of side effects of MAO inhibitors, including dizziness, fainting, headaches, tremors, muscle twitching, confusion, memory impairment, anxiety, agitation, insomnia, weakness, drowsiness, chills, blurred visions, and heart palpitations. Withdrawal from MAO inhibitors should be done very slowly under a doctor's supervision.

Tricyclic Antidepressants

The tricyclics inhibit the uptake of norepinephrine and serotonin and therefore have the same end result as the other two classes of antidepressants, MAO inhibitors and SSRIs. They began to be used in psychiatry in the early 1950s. Imapramine (Tofranil) was one of the first tricyclics and is still one of the most-used medications of the group. Over the years there has been an ongoing development of the other tricyclics, including amitriptyline (Elavil, Endep), desipramine (Norpramine, pertofrane), nortriptyline (Pamelor and Aventyl), trimapramine (Surmontil), protriptyline (Vivactil), doxepin (Adapin, Sinequan), and clomipramine (Anafranil).

The most difficult side effects to cope with are sedation, dry mouth, and impotence. But there are literally a hundred side effects listed in the *Physicians' Desk Reference*, which often cause people to curtail therapy. The side effects are worse than their depression. In the elderly, discontinuation of drug therapy often results in the reoccurrence of depression.

Selective Serotonin Reuptake Inhibitors (SSRIs)

SSRIs inhibit the reuptake of serotonin allowing it to bathe brain neurons for longer periods of time. They also have a similar but lesser effect on two other brain neurotransmitters that affect mood, norepinephrine and dopamine.

Prozac was launched in 1987 and psychiatry or psychiatric patients were never the same. Prozac and its sister medicines boost the levels of the neurotransmitter serotonin in the brain.

Harvard Medical School psychiatrist Joseph Glenmullen, interviewed on April 6, 2000 by the Associated Press, said, "We already know enough to indicate that these drugs should be prescribed far more cautiously." In his book *Prozac Backlash*, Dr. Glenmullen offers dozens of accounts of patients who have suffered antidepressant backlash." Side effects noted by Glenmullen include sexual dysfunction, memory loss, grotesque facial tics, anxiety, and suicidal tendencies. Glenmullen feels that Prozac is toxic to the brain, as was eventually discovered about cocaine, some tranquilizers and other "mood brighteners." Glenmullen also said, "Withdrawal syndromes—which can be debilitating—are estimated to affect up to 50 percent of patients."

The Associated Press warned, "*Prozac Backlash* is packed with footnotes, which could indicate the debate may come to a question of whose studies to believe." They might have also added that it comes down to who funded the studies. "Glenmullen cites studies showing the Prozac class of antidepressants cause sexual dysfunction in up to 60 percent of users." But Eli Lilly, who was very angry with Dr. Glenmullen, countered, "Prozac causes '20 to 30 percent max' of mild to moderate sexual dysfunction. For every footnote he cited showing high rate of sexual dysfunction I can show you the other citations with larger numbers of patients that say just the opposite."

An Associated Press interview with Laura Young, vice president of Community Services for the National Mental Health Association, showed that her fears about *Prozac Backlash* changing people's minds about taking a potentially dangerous medication were elsewhere. She said, "My fear with books like this is it scares people away from getting really important treatment they need...and they may mess around with herbal alternatives."

Dr. Peter Kramer, who wrote *Listening to Prozac* just five years after Prozac hit the market, was intrigued yet skeptical of Prozac because of "its ability to alter personality." He "wondered whether the medication had ironed out too many character-giving wrinkles like overly aggressive plastic surgery." He likened Prozac to "cosmetic psycho-pharmacology." He too wondered how Prozac differs from "amphetamines or cocaine or even alcohol" both in their addictive natures and mood-altering natures.

Dr. Peter R. Breggin, who has been called "the Ralph Nadar of psychiatry," has written several books critical of Prozac, Ritalin, and other psychiatric drugs. Dr. Breggin has practiced psychiatry since 1968. From the outset of his career, Dr. Breggin alerted the medical profession, media, and the public "about the potential dangers of drugs, electroshock, psychosurgery, involuntary treatment, and the biological theories of psychiatry." His first book, *Electroshock: It's Brain-Disabling Effects*, was published in 1979 and exposed the horror and dangers of electroshock therapy for depressed patients.

For thirty years, Dr Breggin has served as a medical expert in many civil and criminal suits including product liability suits against the manufacturers of psychiatric drugs. His work provided the scientific basis for the original combined Prozac suits and for the more recent Ritalin class-action suits.

The Canadian Broadcasting Corporation's *News and*

Current Affairs show did a television documentary in 2001 on the bitter controversy surrounding Dr. David Healy and the Centre for Addiction and Mental Health. The center is one of the country's top research centers and is affiliated with the University of Toronto. The university receives funding from pharmaceutical companies. The documentary said, "Dr. Healy is an expert on antidepressant drugs such as Prozac and the center offered him a prestigious job. But then suddenly it changed its mind. The decision, the critics say, was influenced by the center's relationship with powerful drug companies."

SmithKline Beecham (now GlaxoSmithKline) was sued by relatives of Donald Schell. As reported in the *Guardian*, "The court found that the company's best-selling antidepressant, an SSRI called Seroxat, had caused Schell to murder his wife, daughter, and granddaughter and commit suicide." The *Guardian* interviewed Dr. Healy who said that the company found no increased risk of suicide for depressed people on Seroxat. "But the raw data probably does not support that. Some of the placebo suicides took place while patients were withdrawing from an older drug. When the figures are readjusted without these, they show there is substantially increased risk of suicide on Seroxat." The family was awarded $8 million for their loss.

The Dark Side of Antidepressants

What follows is a list of side effects compiled from peer-reviewed journals. This is a sampling and not a definitive list.

Amitriptyline, Mianserin, and Unilateral ECT: side effects in patients with refractory depression

Antidepressant medication, therapy, and treatment: sexual dysfunction

Benzodiazepines*: inhibit the immune system; disrupts normal sleep; often leads to dependence and abuse; exert an inhibitory function on the immune system; short-term use (diazepam) leads to brief fugue-like state with retrograde amnesia; causes higher risk of cognitive decline especially in the elderly; compromises maximum therapeutic response during a course of unilateral ECT

*Note: **dihydrohonokiol** (a potent anxiolytic compound) does not result in the development of benzodiazepine-like side effects such as motor dysfunction, central depression, amnesia, or physical dependence

Clomipramine: substantial adverse events in the treatment of obsessive-compulsive disorder

Elavil: sleepiness

Electroconvulsive therapy: causes significant headaches in up to 45 percent of patients receiving the treatment; depressive outcome and adverse effects of ECT are independent of age, although older patients have a higher risk of developing dementia; impairment of both verbal and nonverbal functions with bilateral ECT are reported; ECT induced impairments of concentration, short-term memory and learning, and treatment resistant patients were more likely to complain of memory problems six months later; retrograde amnesia follows ECT; visual memory impairment often reported; disorientation increased with the number of treatments; affects regular heart beat; plasma prolactin levels higher following bilateral and unilateral ECT, but they were much higher after bilateral ECT

Estrogen (Premarin): depression in elderly women; no meaningful effect on cognitive performance, dementia severity, behavior, mood and cerebral perfusion in female Alzheimer's disease patients. Therefore, its therapeutic effectiveness is in doubt.

Estrone: a positive correlation between estrone and depression in elderly women

Human Immune Response System: links to the temporal cycles of mood disorders

Imapramine: dry mouth, sweating, and increased heart rate in long-term management of panic disorder with agoraphobia

Immune-inflammatory alterations: dipeptidyl peptidase IV and adenosine deaminase activity decrease in depression

Immune-inflammatory response: increased serum interleukin-1-receptor-antagonist concentrations in major depression

Lithium carbonate: severe aggressive and explosive behavior in younger children more than older children; in aggressive children reports of enuresis, fatigue, ataxia, vomiting, headache, nausea, and stomachache problems

Lorazepam: inappropriate secretions of anti-diuretic hormone

Older antidepressant medications: dry mouth, constipation, dizziness, blurred vision, and tremors

Paxil: dry mouth and constipation; sexual dysfunction

Prozac: severe hyponatremia in elderly patients; inappropriate secretion of antidiuretic hormone in elderly women and in elderly psychiatric patients; interstitial pneumopathy induced; secondary hyperthyroidism; movement disorder; sub-hyaloid hemorrhage; induces anesthesia of vagina and nipples; inappropriate secretion of anti-diuretic hormone; tremors induced; late-onset restlessness, tension, agitation, and sleep disturbances after long-term treatment; acute locomotor effects in young and aged Fischer rats; increases plasma concentrations in SSRI (selective serotonin reuptake inhibitors) and CNS (central nervous system) drug interactions; urinary retention in combination with risperidone; anxiety-like effects in make Sprague-Dawley rats; psychomotor agitation during pharmacotherapy; diarrhea, nausea, insomnia, and headache in patients in general

Psychoneuroimmunology of depression: bio-behavioral interventions to impact psychological adaptation and the course of immune-related disease

SSRI: associated with higher rates of sexual dysfunction; emotional blunting

Tricyclics antidepressants: unacceptable side effects; reoccurrence of unipolar depression in the elderly on discontinuation

Zoloft: sexual problems, anxiety, agitation, headache, nausea, and diarrhea

Dozens of research papers echo the concern about the side effects of SSRIs. The effects of a drug that inhibits potential neurotransmitters can't help but have profound effects on innumerable body functions. Only since their release have we been able to fully document these side effects. Doctors have reported that patients taking Prozac have severe sodium loss, and severe fluid and electrolyte imbalances from inappropriate secretion of antidiuretic hormone (ADH) caused by Prozac.

Prozac also affects different organ systems and can cause interstitial lung disease. There could also be a very real danger of increasing the already high incidence of hypothyroidism with the use of Prozac. Yet, Prozac also causes hyperthyroidism. A bizarre complication of Prozac-induced anesthesia of vagina and nipples implies the drug's interference with female sexual hormones. And sexual dysfunction from SSRIs has led to management protocols, which may or may not include taking another drug such as Viagra.

It appears that no part of the body is left unmolested—even eye hemorrhages have also occurred with the use of Prozac.

Children and adolescents on Prozac have experienced movement disorders, adults have experienced tremors, and animal studies continue to show locomotor side effects with SSRIs.

Drug interactions form another large segment of those patients adversely affected by SSRIs. When other medication is used that has an effect on the brain or central nervous system, there can be negative side effects. One particular drug combination causes urinary retention. Studies are also being done to add drugs to the SSRI protocol to help reduce anxiety, a common side effect. We haven't fully analyzed the side effects of SSRIs, yet it is being given in combination to suppress some of these side effects, which can only lead to more and more complications. And yet another study comparing tricyclics to SSRIs says that SSRIs are very effective for treating anxiety and depression and should be used for patients who suffer from both conditions.

Studying the literature surrounding SSRIs, we find a

flurry of research around depression and the immune system. It appears that the field of psychoneuroimmunology is being overtaken in an attempt to find another class of drugs that will manipulate our immune systems. But what we've learned from our inventory of side effects of antidepressant medication tells us that we are flirting with danger when we make attempts to manipulate any part of our body's complex and unique chemistry.

• CHAPTER 5 •

Alternative Treatments for Body, Nutrition, and Diet

One of the surest ways of 'treating' mild to moderate depression in our society is to help people realize that their feelings of sadness and inadequacy may not be depression at all. Some of these feelings may, in fact, be side effects of advertising. Advertising makes people feel they will lack something or are missing out on something, so they will buy product to make up for that lack. But, it's more pervasive than that; it's as if television and glossy magazines broadcast a way of life that we are made to covet. Kids clamor for toys and a sugarcoated way of life. We are being brainwashed into believing that we need to be happy all the time.

Undiagnosing depression in the majority of people given this label is the best form of therapy. It would also get people off antidepressants and their inevitable and innumerable side effects, which have become an accepted part of drug therapy. It makes sense to avoid those drugs as much as possible. Fortunately, there are many ways to deal with stress and the feelings of depression naturally. Going for a long walk, deep breathing, repeating a positive affirmation, or burning incense, sage, or even tiny amounts of tobacco in the Native American tradition, all lend an air of ritual to your life and allow you time to dialogue with your inner self. Finding a positive connection with your inner self can help to strengthen your resolve and your confidence.

You are what you think you are and you are what you eat. If you eat junk food, you have to put up with junk emotions. Diets loaded with sugar and white flour wreak havoc on your internal chemistry, leading to hypoglycemia and diabetes and emotional imbalance. Processed foods are deficient in the necessary vitamin and mineral co-factors that are required in all metabolic functions of the body. The liver and the nervous system depend on B vitamins and magnesium, to name just two. If these nutrients are deficient, signs of anger, irritability, and anxiety are not far behind.

The research that we've accumulated on diet, nutrition, and alternative modalities for the treatment of depression is vast. It gives you many more choices and options compared to the 'elephant gun' approach of allopathic medicine, which mainly tries to manipulate your neurotransmitters. The more we learn about natural approaches with herbs and nutrients, we find that they too affect neurotransmitters but in a much more subtle and balanced way.

Beyond nutrition, supplements, and herbs, modalities such as electro-acupuncture are noninvasive and have proven to be beneficial in many research trials and have few if any side effects.

Many people when depressed feel unsure about what steps to take. When they see a doctor, they are given certain drug options. But they are not told there are many natural or noninvasive treatments, which don't have the negative side effects of pharmaceuticals.

Chinese medicine practitioners use acupuncture and electro-acupuncture (hooking up acupuncture needles to small electrical currents for greater stimulation) for balancing the body's energy. They don't specifically treat depression but look upon depression as an imbalance. If a patient comes in with a chief complaint of depression, the whole person is assessed. Pulses are taken at the wrist, which indicates what meridians are out of balance; then acupuncture points are put into certain points mapped along the body corresponding to certain lines or "meridians." The result is a shift in energy and relief of symptoms of depression. Perhaps the symptoms of depression were just that, an energy imbalance. In Western terms, they were diagnosed as depressed but responded to the Eastern "art" of medicine, acupuncture.

Challenging the Official Model

When you go to a doctor with few nonspecific symptoms such as fatigue, insomnia, and apathy, you are usually given the label of depression. The doctor may ask some perfunctory questions about stress and tension in your life, to which most people can answer yes, and the diagnosis is made. You may be told that you should learn to relax and slow down, but the easiest and most common treatment of depression is medication.

Not only are your symptoms of fatigue, insomnia, and apathy misdiagnosed but on medication those symptoms are going to be masked by chemicals that manipulate your neurotransmitters. Any symptoms you present the doctor with after the introduction of these drugs will be evidence of your ongoing depression and show the need to increase your medication or add additional antidepressants to the mix.

There are hundreds of diagnosable conditions that are overlooked when fatigue, insomnia, and apathy are misdiagnosed as depression. The following is only a partial list that includes many references to allergies because they produce chemical complexes that affect the brain.

Sugar intolerance causes symptoms of hypoglycemia and prediabetes that can go undiagnosed. A gluten allergy from rye, oats, wheat, and barley causes particular chemicals to affect the brain. Some people are allergic to dairy products and the resulting intestinal flora imbalance leads to brain allergy symptoms. Similarly, a mold allergy from various foods including peanuts and two-day-old leftovers, a mold allergy from tobacco, and a mold allergy from mildew in your home can cause mental and emotional symptoms that some people misinterpret as depression. An allergy to fermented foods, such as beverages including alcohol, can cause emotional symptoms as can sensitivity to hundreds of additives, dyes, colorings, and preservatives in our food and beverages.

Artificial hormones injected into beef and poultry can affect meat, dairy, and eggs and pass on allergenic triggers that affect the nervous system. In fact, an allergy, sensitivity, or poisoning can occur from one or more chemicals in our air, food, or water including fluoride, choline, pesticides, and herbicides, which can affect the brain. Heavy metal poisoning with mercury, lead, and arsenic all have a well-known history of causing symptoms from mental retardation to insanity.

The *Physicians' Desk Reference* lists hundreds of prescription drugs with the side effect of emotional instability and depression. Depression is also common in the face of vitamin, mineral, amino acid, and essential fatty acid deficiencies. None of these deficiencies are studied carefully in hospital settings for doctors to develop an appreciation of how important nutrients are to mental health. Even simple hormonal deficiencies such as adrenal insufficiency, thyroid hormone deficiency, and DHEA deficiency along with the more common estrogen, progesterone, and testosterone deficiencies are mostly overlooked by busy doctors who still view the mind and body as separate.

There are many infectious causes of depression. We know that viral hepatitis can cause mental instability, and the same can be said for chronic fungal (Candida) and parasitic infections. Inflammatory bowel disease, whether caused by infection or food allergy, causes punctures in the lining of the intestines, which allow incompletely broken down food molecules to enter the blood and act as allergens.

We also want to show you that misdiagnosis is very common in everyday medical practice when the medical model, based on scientific proof, is applied to many other diseases.

During the past century, a medical establishment has evolved that has made itself the exclusive provider of so-called scientific, evidence-based therapies. The paradigm used by this establishment is what we call the orthodox medical approach, and for the first 70 years of this century, little effort was made to challenge it. In the past 30 years, however, there has been a growing awareness of the importance of an alternative approach to medical care, one that, either on its own or as a complement to orthodox medicine, emphasizes nontoxic and noninvasive treatments and prevention.

Unfortunately, this new perspective has been fought vigorously. We've been told that it's only the treatments of orthodox medicine that have passed careful scientific scrutiny involving double-blind, placebo-controlled studies. Concomitantly, we've been told that alternative or complementary health care has no science to back it up, only anecdotal evidence. These two ideas have led to widely accepted "truths": anyone offering an alternative or complementary approach is depriving patients of the proven benefits of safe and effective care, and people don't get well with alternative care but are actually endangered by it.

By getting society to accept these precepts, orthodox medicine has maneuvered itself into becoming the sole provider of information about disease and its treatment and has taken charge of curricula, accreditation, and insurance coverage in the health care arena. All 50 states have enacted strict standards at the state medical board level against using so-called unscientific medicine, meaning anything that is not, according to orthodox consensus, common-use medicine. Many physicians have been prosecuted and punished for not confining their treatments to the accepted paradigm, some to the point of having their licenses revoked, being imprisoned, or suffering bankruptcy. And it has been only of secondary importance whether or not their patients have claimed to benefit from their treatments. The prosecutors—the state attorneys general working hand-in-hand with state medical boards and "anti-quackery" groups supported by pharmaceutical interests—have influenced such federal enforcement agencies as the FDA, the USDA, and the Department of Justice. They've also influenced such bodies as the National Institutes of Health as to which modalities receive funding and get incorporated into the standard medical model, thus perpetuating the status quo.

It is the purpose of this review to question the status quo. Specifically, we'll be looking at a variety of areas—cancer, heart disease, mental illness, obstetrics and gynecology, psychiatry, etc.—and asking some basic questions:

1. Are the orthodox medical modalities safe and effective, i.e., have they been proven so by qualified science?

2. If they have not been proven safe and effective, then what are the risk/benefit ratios of using these modalities?

3. What are the costs, in terms of morbidity and mortality, as well as dollars and cents, of using these modalities, both to the individual and society?

After a careful consideration of the answers, we can determine how much of the existing mainstream medical model should be rejected and replaced with new approaches.

It is vital to note that all the studies referred to here are from mainstream medicine's own respected journals such as the *Journal of the American Medical Association* (*JAMA*), the *New England Journal of Medicine*, and *The Lancet*. Thus the book's criticism of the various therapies comes not from the "alternative" world, but from the very heart of orthodox medicine itself and from researchers using the gold standard of rigorously set-up and controlled studies. So there is nothing subjective or political about the conclusions. Also, I should mention that this work was done over a period of eight years, during which time more than a thousand of studies were analyzed. The studies contained herein are just a sample; many more could have been included but were not because of a consideration of length.

With thousands of physicians questioned, it is apparent that the vast majority of medical procedures are done with the belief that they are safe and effective rather than with proof that they are. Even after procedures and medications have been shown (a) not only not to work, but (b) to cause injury and death at a statistically significant level, they continue to gain in popularity and use. This is one of the reasons we have not had greater gains in combating the major diseases in recent decades. And it is also why there is an urgent need for physicians, legislators, journalists, funding agencies, curriculum developers, insurance companies, and peer-review systems to take note of the substantial gaps in primary chronic care and find better approaches.

The facts here speak for themselves. We are a society that states that we live by the gold standard of scientific research, but we are routinely causing iatrogenic conditions and unnecessary suffering, not to mention wasting vast sums of money, through a systematic negligence of the facts. This situation must be challenged and remedied. So look at the facts we present herein. It may be tedious, but the facts must carry the day.

But why are we challenging the standard medical model?

Because patients with depression and anxiety are not aware of the consequences of an incorrect diagnosis. We will show that it can be lethal. By presenting just a random review of the application of this model to other diseases, the reader can see that there is a larger pattern of misdiagnosis that carries over to the diagnosis of depression and anxiety. And the problem is in the general model. You don't believe us? The *BMJ* published an article in 2000 that reviewed the incidence and nature of medical errors in U.S. hospitals and found that 48,000–98,000 patients were killed each year and an additional 1 million were injured. To determine the incidence of adverse drug reactions, they reviewed the patients' medical charts and conducted interviews with physicians. They found that 6.5 percent of hospitalized patients developed an adverse drug reaction and another 5.5 percent developed a potential adverse drug reaction; these events were found to be caused by errors in 28 percent of the cases. Another study calculated that every year, treatment-related complications result in 116 million additional physicians visits, 76 million prescriptions, 17 million emergency room visits, 8 million hospital admissions, 3 million long-term care facility admissions, and 200,000 additional deaths, for a cost of $76.6 billion. These data, however, significantly underestimate the real extent of the problem, since they only refer to hospital patients and are not inclusive of errors occurring in nursing homes and other health care settings. Another article in the *BMJ* questioned some of the data that emerged from two studies conducted by the Institute of Medicine showing that, every year, approximately 100,000 patients die needlessly in the hospital as a result of errors in medical management, and many more are injured. And the article added that 50–96 percent of adverse events are not reported. It concluded that preventable deaths from errors in medical management have reached endemic proportions, and that the extent of the injuries is largely underestimated.

The reason for many of the iatrogenic mistakes is that the research the standard model claims is "scientific" is not so at all. In 1994 an article published in the *BMJ* questioned the integrity of the medical research community, pointing out those responsible for the production and the publication of scientific articles in which statistical analysis is often misused, studies are poorly designed, results are misinterpreted and selectively reported, and unjustified conclusions are drawn. It emphasized that all of the above phenomena are frequently found in medical literature and are due to the pressure placed on physicians to publish in order to advance their careers. The consequences of the poor quality research can be devastating, especially since patient treatment is often based on trial results, which can be statistically manipulated to show the safety and effectiveness of a specific treatment. The article concluded that "there may be greater danger to the public welfare from statistical dishonesty than from almost any other form of dishonesty." In 1999 another *BMJ* article highlighted that trials supported by pharmaceutical companies are significantly more likely to report favorable outcomes associated with the use of the sponsored drug, compared to non-sponsored trials. Beside the unscientific milieu that produces flawed treatments, iatrogenic problems arise because the unproven treatments, usually pharmaceutical, enter the doctors' offices through dubious conflicts of interest. In 2000 *JAMA* published a study that indicated that pharmaceutical companies significantly influence physicians' professional behavior through gifts, free meals, sponsored travels, teaching seminars, and symposia.

It found that every year the pharmaceutical industry spends more than $12 billion to push drugs and invests an estimated $8,000 to $13,000 on each U.S. physician. While 85 percent of medical students believed that politicians accepting gifts is unethical, only 46 percent of them believed that it is improper to accept a gift of similar value themselves from a pharmaceutical company. The article concluded that "the interaction between physicians and the drug industry could have crucial consequences if it can be demonstrated that such relationship results in changes in prescribing practices toward drugs that are more expensive or that are associated with negative health outcomes." The *BMJ* is not waiting for such a "demonstration" because it published an article in 1999 that referred to studies on the contact between doctors and drug companies' sales representatives, which demonstrated that the more doctors rely on information from drug company representatives, the less rational their prescribing is. There are strong reasons for physicians not being allowed to see pharmaceutical representatives.

The drug companies' influence is not only corrupting the studies that are being published in supposedly "scientific" journals. Now the journals themselves are becoming compromised. A study alleged that medical organizations are increasingly becoming dependent on the drug industry for their income, which can pose a threat to their objectivity. The study evaluated the profits of the clinical journals of several leading medical organizations including the *Journal of the American Medical Association,* the *New England Journal of Medicine,* the *Journal of the American College of Cardiology, Annals of Internal Medicine, Clinical Infectious Diseases,* and others. Drug advertisements contributed from $715,000 to $18 million of revenue, a sum that, according to the study, could place the organization in a position of dependency. The study also revealed that more than 10 percent of the income of five medical organizations came from drug advertisements published in a single journal, while four organizations profited as much or more from drug advertisements as they did from subscriptions.

Meanwhile, as the hoax of the "scientific" foundations for modern medicine increasingly unravels, the disastrous consequences from iatrogenic errors are becoming more obvious. Patients in chronic care need to be extremely cautious while listening to their physicians, even during the established procedures for diagnosis. An article in 1996 emphasized that 60 percent of routine tests conducted on patients in preparation for surgery were unnecessary and added an extra $18 billion to the annual health care bill. In addition, unnecessary tests caused harm resulting from complications associated with the testing procedure, or with the unnecessary treatment of patients who received a false positive test result. A 1993 study reviewed all relevant articles published in English, French, and Spanish from 1966 to 1992, and concluded that the costs of routine chest X rays are so high and the benefits so small, that its use is no longer justified in patients who have received a careful analysis and clinical evaluation. In a particular study of fetal occult blood screening for colorectal neoplasia conducted on over 13,000 individuals, Ahlquist et al. found that two of the most widely used tests for the detection of colorectal cancer, the Hemoccult and Hemoquant tests, missed approximately 70 percent of cancers that were later diagnosed by other methods and 90 percent of polyps (precancerous conditions) 1 centimeter or more in size.

Once the patient surmounts the hurdles blocking an accurate diagnosis, there are also the dangers of predominant treatments that have not been properly studied. The use of nonsteroidal anti-inflammatory drugs (NSAIDs) can cause hospitalization for congestive heart failure in individuals with or without a history of heart disease. Heart failure affects approximately 4.6 million Americans, and this condition represents the most common hospital discharge diagnosis among patients older than 65 years. If this association is causal as the dose-response relation suggests, cardiovascular morbidity due to NSAIDs would surpass gastrointestinal NSAID-related morbidity, which alone is responsible for a minimum of 105,000 hospitalizations and 24,000 deaths each year in the U.S. The economic and health consequences for these findings are staggering.

A study presented at the American College of Cardiology's 49th annual scientific meeting held in California showed that hormone replacement therapy has no beneficial effects on the cardiovascular system. The study was conducted on 309 postmenopausal women with coronary heart disease who were randomly assigned to receive one of the three treatments: estrogen, estrogen plus progestin, or placebo. No differences in disease progression were observed between the three groups, suggesting that neither estrogen alone nor estrogen combined with a progestin, offer protection to women from heart disease. A second study compared the effects of hormone replacement therapy, placebo, no therapy, or vitamins on the incidence of cardiovascular diseases. The results in the analysis indicated that women who took hormones had a 40 percent increased risk of cardiovascular events other than pulmonary embolism and deep vein thrombosis, and a 64 percent increased risk of cardiovascular events including venous thromboembolism, compared to women who did not take hormones. These results are in contrast with the commonly held assumption that hormone replacement therapy prevents cardiovascular diseases. Yet hormone replacement therapy is widely prescribed for American women. Also, many American women are routinely advised to take birth control pills, but have their doctors told them of a recent study, conducted on 46,000 women who were followed up with over a period of 25 years, that demonstrated that users of oral contraceptives have a 2.5 times increased risk of death of cancer of the uterine cervix, a twofold increased risk of death from cerebrovascular diseases, and a fivefold increased risk of death from liver cancer, compared to nonusers? The study also found that the adverse effects persisted for 10 years after the interruption of oral contraceptives intake and ceased afterwards. Yet the common assumption is that the use of oral contraceptives is associated with an 80 percent decreased risk of death from ovarian cancer. Another study showed that women of childbearing age using combined oral contraceptives had an almost tenfold risk of dying from pulmonary embolism, compared to nonusers. The finding of a substantial increased risk of this fatal complication in users of oral contraceptives is especially important when considering that these deaths occur in healthy young women who would have otherwise had a long life ahead of them. Now women who want to have children suffer the same iatrogenic effects as those avoiding childbirth if they listen to their doctor. Almost 10 years ago, a study conducted on a sample population of 3,837 women who received fertility drugs found that the use of these drugs is associated with a 2.4 times increased risk of invasive or borderline ovarian cancer, compared to nonuse. Once the pregnant American woman is giving birth, another problem surfaces: in the U.S., almost one out of four deliveries made is performed by Cesarean section. These rates are among the highest recorded in developed countries. From 1970 to 1993, overall rates of primary Cesarean sections of primary Cesarean sections increased fourfold, from 5.5 percent to 22.8 percent. Deliveries by Cesarean sections carry a significantly higher risk of complications for both the mother and the newborn. Another study done about the same time highlighted how decisions concerning the need for Cesarean delivery seem to be influenced by more social, economic, and physicians' personal reasons than by medical factors. This is well illustrated by the fact that those women who are at highest risk of pregnancy complications and who would benefit the most from a Cesarean section are the least likely to receive it. On the other hand, indications such as previous Cesarean, slow or difficult labor or delivery, presentation of the rear of the baby at the uterine cervix, and fetal distress are the main reasons for performing a C-section, even though these conditions have been at least clearly associated with benefits for the fetus and the mother.

    Now let's look at prevalent health problems and note the

side effects of established treatments supposedly backed up by scientific standards. A recent study showed that asthma patients receiving ipratropium bromide and theophylline have an 80 percent and threefold increased risk of death from respiratory causes, respectively, compared to those taking salmeterol. All three drugs are regularly used for patients with asthma of increasing severity. And an earlier study showed that the trend of prescribing corticosteroids as anti-inflammatory drugs for adult asthma (to a growing number of patients in larger doses and for longer periods of time) has been associated with an increased rate of potentially serious systematic adverse reactions such as adrenal suppression, osteoporosis, cataract, stunted growth in children, altered metabolism, and behavioral abnormalities. Reviewing the studies on treatments for cancer we find the same failures of modern claims. A study in 1997 showed that U.S. cancer mortality rates in 1994 were 6 percent higher than in 1970. Cancer mortality rates increased steadily for nearly two decades, reached a plateau, and then decreased by 1 percent from 1991 to 1994. The authors of the study said this decrease can be attributed to a reduction in cigarette smoking and early detection, but not to the effects of new treatments, which have been largely disappointing. The authors concluded, "35 years of intense effort focused largely on improving treatment must be judged a qualified failure," and argued that progress can occur only through a national commitment to prevention through reallocation of funding and shift of research focus.

In another article, Frezza et al. reviewed all cases of gallbladder cancer treated at Howard University during the last 20 years to determine the efficacy of nonsurgical therapies. No improved survival was observed in patients treated with chemotherapy or radiotherapy. Nor on gastric cancer, esophageal cancer, head and neck cancer, lung cancer, melanoma, pancreatic cancer, renal cancer, nor uterine cancer. And moving along to diabetes, we have a study that shows intensive treatment of type 2 diabetic patients with sulphonylureas or insulin, compared to conventional treatment (consisting of diet with the addition of pharmacological treatment if glucose levels cannot be controlled by diet alone), decreases the risk of microvascular complications (i.e., retinopathy, nephropathy, and neuropathy) but has no effect in preventing macrovascular complications. Furthermore, patients in the intensive treatment group experienced significantly more hypoglycemic episodes and weight gain compared to those in the standard treatment group. Weight gain was especially high in patients treated with insulin. Standard antiepileptic drugs don't work either, as D. Chadwick showed in his 1995 survey where a randomized trial by Temkin et al. was conducted on a cohort of patients with seizures following head injury. Individuals taking the antiepileptic drug phenytoin experienced more seizures than those receiving placebo. As the author concludes, "None of the available clinical trials comparing early treatment with deferred treatment seemed to show any great doubts on the value of early treatment for epilepsy." Finally, be forewarned of the dangers of a hospital stay. In 2000 an article reported that every year in the U.S. approximately two million patients develop hospital-acquired infections and 88,000 die from them. The cost of hospital-acquired infections has been estimated at $4 to 6 billion. These estimates are conservative, because they do not take into account nosocomial infections occurring in patients in nursing homes, outpatient clinics, dialysis centers, and other health care centers.

There are countries such as Germany and Italy that use intravenous ozone post-operatively to lessen infections and save patients lives. We are not yet that progressive in the United States.

• CHAPTER 6 •

Comparing Orthodox Versus Alternative Therapies and Their Outcomes

Virginia Woolf, Ernest Hemingway, Michelangelo, and Gustav Mahler. What did they have in common, other than their great talents? They all suffered from what author Andrew Solomon very appropriately called "The Noon-Day Demon": depression.

Dr. Jay Lombard, board-certified neurologist, former chief of Neurology at Westchester Square Medical Center, and author of *The Brain Wellness Plan*, puts depression at the top of the list of modern epidemics. According to Dr. Lombard, 20 percent of adults in the U.S. experience one or more depressive episodes, while 5 percent receive a diagnosis of clinical depression. Of the latter group, 15 percent of the cases end in suicide.

An especially alarming trend is the increase of incidence of depression among teens and young adults, and even children. Statistics show that an average of 14 teens kill themselves every day. That's 5,000 kids a year. It is estimated that 5 percent of American teenagers currently suffer from depression severe enough to warrant medical treatment, but these numbers may not reflect a much more alarming reality.

It is no surprise, given these statistics, that pharmaceutical companies are so eager to fund research aimed at finding effective relief for this life-threatening condition. And yet, current drug treatment seems to fall short of expectations. It works sometimes, for some people, but for many, it becomes a frustrating juggling act from one drug to another, waiting for an elusive relief that never seems to come or never seems to stay.

And while the initial lessening of symptoms offered by antidepressants is desirable and necessary, it carries the potential for serious, long-term, undesirable side effects such as tardive diskenesia, paranoid and psychotic reactions, and liver malfunctions, among others.

Candace B. Pert, Ph.D., is mostly known for her discovery of endorphins, the opiate-like chemicals produced by the brain and nervous system. Her pioneering work has led the way into this quickly expanding field of research and has been one of the most important foundations for establishing the biomolecular connection between brain chemistry and emotional states.

Experts may disagree on how to treat depression, but there is almost unanimous consent that depression is caused by a chemical imbalance in the flow of the neurotransmitters that bathe our brains at any given moment—too much of one or not enough of another. All it takes is a rebalancing act, research seems to promise. The task of the health care practitioner, according to this approach, lies in figuring out which chemical or chemicals are out of balance and to provide the patient with a drug that corrects the problem. If it sounds too simple to be true, than it probably is. And it's the best current psychiatry has to offer.

To challenge the axiom that the patient's brain chemistry is inherently faulty and therefore in need of permanent outside intervention, we decided to conduct our own study using alternative methods. In other words, we changed the therapeutic stance from one that defines the patient as a passive, helpless victim of a fateful brain dysfunction to one that puts him or her in the driver seat of this delicate and possibly lifesaving "brain rescue" operation.

The results of our study, we are delighted to say, have opened a window of hope for those who suffer from this very painful and often devastating condition. Indeed, we believe that this remarkable study, unique in its parameters, offers a new foundation upon which to build the future of brain research.

We didn't try to forcibly redirect brain chemistry by supplementing the participants' diet with isolated nutrients and/or herbal supplements, nor did we require that participants stop taking their medications prescribed for their symptoms. Rather, our aim was to find out whether neurotransmitter imbalances leading to depression could be the consequence of lifestyle choices—not an elusive brain abnormality that can only be affected by aggressive chemical interventions.

To establish whether or not this was true or not, we designed a parallel study where participants were given high doses of nutrients known to positively affect brain functioning such as St. John's wort, PS and PC complexes, SAMe, DHA, and others. No other change was required—dietary or otherwise. The outcome of this study showed that single, isolated nutrients have little or no impact on mental outlook and overall health. Symptoms of anxiety and/or depression persisted. And no major positive change was noted in this group.

Participants in the first group ranged from 20 to 78 years old. In order to be accepted in to the study, all of the participants had to present a letter from their physician stating that they had been diagnosed with, and were in treatment for, anxiety and/or depression, primary or secondary. If they were taking nutritional supplements on their own, such as a multivitamin or a B-complex, we asked them to suspend supplementation for the duration of the study. However, we told them to continue taking their medications as prescribed by their doctor. All medical aspects of the study were closely monitored by Martin Feldman, M.D., a board-certified neurologist.

The need for lifestyle modification was discussed and explained in detail to the participant and attendance to weekly meetings was made mandatory, in order to effectively monitor the evolution of the study. All of them were asked to implement the following changes:

1. Identify and eliminate all known allergens or toxins from the diet. Plus learn to purchase, prepare, and enjoy good, healthy, and natural foods.

2. Self-administer a simple test in order to evacuate thyroid activity.

3. Establish, maintain, and gradually increase intake of beneficial phytochemicals from fresh vegetables and fruit juices and/or from food concentrates.

4. Avoid watching television, except for movie classics and educational programs. We also asked that participants refrain from reading upsetting news for obvious reasons.

5. Learn stress management tools such as relaxation, meditation, prayer, positive affirmations, and positive thinking techniques. Use them daily for the minimum of an hour.

6. Engage in one hour of mild to moderate daily aerobic exercises as well as learn basic yoga and breathing techniques.

7. Identify and correct hormonal imbalances, especially for men and women whose hormonal status may be one of the major underlying causes of brain imbalances (i.e., reduced testosterone, imbalanced thyroid, etc.).

8. And finally, perhaps most importantly, we encouraged participants to do whatever was necessary to boost and restore efficacious immunity. For many of them, one of the greatest discoveries was linking mercury amalgam fillings in their teeth with their mental anguish; once the mercury was removed, many of the gloomy feelings seemed to disappear as well.

Once the relevance of the required change was understood, its implementation was facilitated and made possible by providing participants with simple, practical information and support at our weekly meetings. These meetings lasted two hours and offered an open forum for individuals to share their experience with one another, thereby creating an opportunity for positive reinforcement of their newly learned behaviors. We also provided individual counseling and support as needed.

After three months on the program, without heavy-duty nutritional or herbal intervention, 93 percent of participants reported markedly elevated energy level, relief of anxiety and depression symptoms, improved cognition, better sleep, improvement in digestion and elimination, better focusing ability, and a sense of internal peace and confidence as well as significant improvement in overall mental state.

Many felt confident enough to ask their physician to lessen or discontinue their medication and thus were able to sustain a stable, drug-free, comfortable lifestyle. What was especially remarkable was that, along with the subsiding of anxiety and depression symptoms, all participants across the board achieved a level of overall health they had not been able to achieve or sustain previously.

We hope that this study will serve as a template for future research, and we present it in this book as a prototype for what we consider a state-of-the-art approach to the treatment of anxiety and depression.

Food Sensitivities, Diet, Neurotoxins, and Brain Health

Our modern diet is conveniently suited for a fast-paced lifestyle—one that emphasizes productivity at the expense of quality. When we consume highly processed foods, fast foods, soft drinks, caffeinated beverages, and alcohol (in any form), we may temporarily experience a surge of artificial energy and may be misled into believing that our brain's nutritional needs have been met. However, nothing could be further from the truth. The artificial stimulation that enables us to be more productive eventually takes a heavy toll on our health, possibly establishing the groundwork for depression and anxiety to take hold.

Even though people have unique allergy profiles determined by the individual's history and set of circumstances, some popular food items and drinks seem to cause allergic reactions in most people. These items include products containing sugar and gluten, caffeinated and alcoholic drinks, artificial sweeteners, hydrogenated fats, cold cuts, and other processed meats, food containing MSG (monosodium glutamate) and/or other flavor enhancers, preservatives, and artificial color. We asked the participants in one study to abstain from these items and to avoid nicotine (in any form) as well as recreational substances, legal or illegal.

In order to establish and correct individual allergies, we then taught participants two of the simplest methods of self-assessment. The first method requires that one abstain from a suspected food item for a week, then consume a considerable amount of the same food all at once. If an unusual reaction occurs, or if there is a flare-up of symptoms that had temporarily subsided, chances argue the food is allergenic for that individual.

In the other method, the food in question is eliminated from the diet, again, for one week. On the morning of the eighth day, one's pulse should be taken upon awakening, before getting up or doing anything else. After mentally recording this initial reading, the person is instructed to swallow a small piece of the food and lay in bed for twenty minutes. The heart rate is then checked again. If a five beats-per-minute increase is noted, the food is most likely causing an allergic reaction and should be removed from the diet, at least temporarily.

Avoiding potentially neurotoxic and allergy-causing foods is an absolute necessity, since their metabolic by-products have the capacity to interfere with normal brain functions. Because so many staples in the standard American diet fall into this category, participants in this study were given instructions on how to buy fresh, organic, and nonallergenic food items. They were also given recipes and explanations of how to cook these foods and prepare delicious, wholesome, vegetarian meals with the inclusion of some fish and organic poultry, if desired.

A very strong emphasis was placed on drinking freshly extracted vegetable juices, starting with one glass a day for the first week of the study and increasing by one glass each subsequent week, until total juice intake reached two quarts per day, after which it was maintained at that level. To those participants suffering from diabetes, who could not negotiate the fructose in juices, we showed how to obtain the same beneficial effects by taking fruit and vegetable concentrates from which the fructose had been removed.

These comprehensive dietary changes did bring on the results we had hoped for, namely, a gradual and steady decrease in symptoms of anxiety and depression, as we reported above, in 93 percent of the participants. They also brought on several desirable side effects such as more stable glucose blood levels, improvement of cardiovascular health, weight loss or gain reflective of improved assimilation and metabolism, pain relief for those suffering from arthritis and other chronic inflammatory conditions, not to mention better memory, clearer thinking, and increased libido.

Stress Management

We are constantly taking in our environment in the form of cosmic dust, floating microorganisms, and other microscopic particles, sounds, sights, aromas, magnetic waves, and information affecting our psyche. When we focus on something, we increase our "attentional" intake of that particular object, thereby increasing its potential impact on our psychic structure. This is how we create mental landscape, where memory, imagination, and perception join together to give us a sense of what our reality is really like.

In other words, what we selectively absorb from our environment determines, to a large extent, how we feel about being in it. If we allow our ears to be flooded with news of death and destruction all day long, our brain may eventually become accustomed to high levels of neurotransmitters that spell disaster in response to what we perceive.

This kind of habitual, negative input can affect brain chemistry and aggravate symptoms of anxiety and depression. So can excessive, up-close TV watching, simply as a result of magnetic waves. For the reasons mentioned above, the first step in establishing a successful stress management strategy was for participants to abstain from watching TV or reading newspapers.

Removing potentially distressing negative input was the first step in the stress management component of our study. We guided the participants to use many well-known, simple, and effective self-help techniques including yoga and deep breathing, relaxation, meditation, visualization, positive affirmations, prayer, self-hypnosis, bio-feedback, tai chi and qigong, among others. We recommended engaging in any of these activities, according to individual preferences, for at least an hour a day.

Instructions on how to safely engage in mild to moderate aerobic exercise, for a least one hour a day, was the third and final element included in the stress management part of the study. As a result of this comprehensive approach, we believe the positive changes brought on by an improved nutritional status were potentiated and reinforced, thereby creating powerful synergistic dynamic between mind and body.

This newfound sense of well-being served to increase rewarding inner feelings such as a sense of peace and self-confidence. Participants felt that what they were getting out of the study was well worth the efforts required in order to participate in it.

Heart disease and clinical depression present with different symptoms and are conventionally managed with different treatments. While heart disease can be very life threatening, depression tends to be slow and develops over time. How can the conditions of heart disease and depression be possibly related?

Depression and Heart Disease

Emerging research indicates that the deeper we probe, the more alike the two disorders appear to be. While the ultimate manifestations of heart disease and depression differ, the underlying biochemical pathologies are surprisingly similar. Beneath the emotional surface of mood and depression can be a raging physical undercurrent of hormonal distortions, impaired immunity, and inflammation. These disturbances of physiology contribute to the growth and abnormal activity of coronary plaque, eventually leading to heart attack. Depressed people, in fact, suffer a fourfold greater risk of heart attack compared to non-depressed people.

If the two seemingly disparate disorders of depression

and coronary heart disease share common causes, can there also be common treatments? Exciting new insights suggest that strategies to address both conditions do exist. These therapies work by treating the shared metabolic origins of heart disease and depression. The good news is that some of these treatments are powerful nutritional therapeutics, readily available to all.

Depression: More than a Feeling

Everyone has had the experience of feeling sad or blue. How do these everyday feelings differ from clinical depression? Symptoms of depression include loss of interest in activities one previously enjoyed, struggling to sleep or awakening early, difficulty concentrating, feelings of worthlessness or guilt, loss of appetite or weight, and suicidal thoughts. Symptoms that interfere with daily activities and that last longer than two weeks may signal clinical depression.

Far more than just a state of mind involving sadness or hopelessness, depression is a disease in the true organic sense, with measurable symptoms. In the last decade, clinical investigations have uncovered the myriad physical manifestations of depression. Until recently, these manifestations have been little understood, but growing evidence asserts that they have very real consequences.

Feeling good can hinge on a precarious balance of internal dialogue and external events. This balance can easily tip, setting the stage for negative emotions and the resulting metabolic consequences. At what point do negative emotions begin to add to the risk for heart disease?

The line that separates depression from the more commonplace feelings of sadness and anger, which are part of all our lives, can be somewhat hazy. It is a matter of the degree and duration of symptoms. Full-blown depression is not necessary to increase your risk of heart disease; even moderate feelings of hopelessness and sadness can more than double the risk of heart attack. People who chronically experience negative emotions—unexpressed anger, hostility, and resentment—also have a higher risk for heart attack. They experience a level of risk similar to that of fully depressed people.

Metabolic Underpinnings of Depression

Beneath the surface of sadness and hopelessness blazes an inferno of metabolic phenomena. Increased levels of inflammatory proteins such as interleukin-1 beta (IL-1b) and tumor necrosis factor alpha (TNF-a) circulate in the blood, suggesting that low-grade, body-wide inflammation accompanies depression. IL-1b and TNF-a levels correlate with the severity of depression, with higher levels of inflammatory proteins linked to more serious depression. C-reactive protein is another inflammatory protein found at higher levels in depressed individuals. All these inflammatory mediators have been clearly linked to increased risk of heart attack. Extensive clinical trial data show that when the fires of inflammation are burning, coronary plaque is unstable and more prone to "rupture," an event that can lead to heart attacks.

Just as a life-threatening event such as a car accident triggers biochemical reactions in the body, depression activates the release of stress hormones. The feelings of anger, frustration, hostility, and anxiety are also associated with increased levels of stress hormones. Hypersecretion of the corticotrophin-releasing hormone from the hypothalamus triggers the release of cortisol and norepinephrine, both of which are involved in the survival response that occurs when the human organism is threatened. These hormones are potent contributors to hypertension, insulin resistance, and diabetes, three well-established risks for coronary disease.

When negative emotions become chronic and deeply rooted, the risk for developing pathological heart disease grows.

Cortisol and norepinephrine also contribute to development of metabolic syndrome, which is a combination of abdominal obesity, hypertension, low high-density lipoprotein (HDL), and higher blood sugar (above 110 mg/dL). The epidemic numbers of overweight and obese people in America are fueling a skyrocketing increase in metabolic syndrome, estimated to currently affect 47 million adults in the U.S. Metabolic syndrome is a rapidly growing cause of heart disease, and depressed people are particularly prone to develop the features of metabolic syndrome.

During periods of depression, the "fight-or-flight" response of the sympathetic nervous system operates in a continuous state of heightened activation, releasing stress hormones into the bloodstream. The calming parasympathetic system is simultaneously suppressed. This reaction can be measured as blunted, beat-to-beat variation in heart rate, or heart-rate variability, even when the heart rate is normal. Decreased heart-rate variability predicts heightened potential for dangerous heart (ventricular) arrhythmias and sudden death.

For years, epidemiologists have explored the unexpectedly low risk of both heart disease and depression in cultures in which fish is eaten in abundant quantities. The common thread seems to be the high content of omega-3 fatty acids in fish oils. Through his studies across numerous cultures, Dr. Joseph Hibbeln of the National Institutes of Health has documented the remarkable association between higher levels of fish consumption and lower rates of depression. He was also among the first to draw the connection between greater fish consumption and the lower likelihood of heart attack.

Indeed, both depression and heart disease are associated with low concentrations of omega-3 fatty acids in red blood cells. Conventional prescription antidepressant medication fails to correct an imbalance of omega-3 fatty acids. It is tempting to suggest that supplementation with fish oil rich in omega-3 fatty acids might provide a common therapy for both depression and heart disease. Research discussed later in this chapter suggests that it does.

Homocysteine represents another intriguing connection between depression and heart disease. Homocysteine, an amino acid associated with the deficiency of certain B vitamins, has been clearly and conclusively associated with increased risk of heart attack. Less well known is homocysteine's role in emotions. Depression, poor response to antidepressant medication, and dysthymia (a lesser form of depression) have all been linked to low blood levels of folic acid. Folic acid deficiency causes high homocysteine blood levels. Folate-deficient people are also more likely to be deeply depressed and for longer periods. Up to 50 percent of depressed people have homocysteine levels that are significantly above normal, which is considered to be greater than 10 micromoles per liter (µmol/L) of blood. This variety of depression responds poorly to antidepressant medication but does respond to folic acid. Studies examining depressed people in a number of settings have firmly established that folic acid replacement, resulting in reduced homocysteine blood levels, is an effective treatment for depression and a useful addition to prescription antidepressant therapies.

Depression and feelings of anger, hostility, and anxiety share several biochemical traits that are similar to those that form the foundations of risk for heart disease. These include a tendency toward inflammation, increased levels of stress hormones, the presence of metabolic syndrome, blunted heart-rate variability, reduced levels of omega-3 fatty acids, and elevated homocysteine levels. Nutritional supplements may be powerful tools in managing the overlapping syndromes of depression and heart disease.

To help lower your homocysteine levels:

N-acetylcysteine. This supplement can lower your homocysteine levels through raising cysteine production, which in turn assists in the production of glutathione. Glutathione is integral in many metabolic and biochemical reactions and helps in protein synthesis, DNA synthesis and repair, amino acid transport, and enzyme activation, so every system in your body can benefit from N-acetylcysteine. And if you body is functioning better, so can you.

Creatine. If you supplement with SAMe, more than half will be utilized in the synthesis of creatine. Consuming creatine lowers the need for SAMe and lowers homocysteine production as well as the need for homocysteine remethylation.

The Omega-3 Connection

Fish oil, containing abundant quantities of the omega-3 fatty acids docosahexaenoic acid (DHA) and eicosapentaenoic acid (EPA), is a dual-action supplement with compelling data to support its use for both depression and heart disease. Some have called omega-3 fatty acids the "missing link" between the two disorders.

The human brain contains an extraordinarily high concentration of omega-3 fatty acids. This simple fact has prompted extensive investigation of the role of essential fats in various brain functions and diseases. A deficiency of omega-3 fatty acids has been associated with conditions as diverse as hostility, cognitive decline with aging, and attention-deficit/hyperactivity disorder. Several studies have demonstrated that people suffering from major depression are measurably deficient in omega-3 fatty acids. Not surprisingly, these and other studies have highlighted the failure of conventional antidepressant medication to correct the omega-3 deficiency. From an epidemiological viewpoint, cultures marked by abundant fish consumption and omega-3 intake, for example, Eskimos and some of the coastal natives of Japan and Canada, are far less likely to suffer from depression than Americans. Conversely, cultures consuming less fish than Americans, like New Zealanders, suffer substantially higher rates of depression.

An ultra low-fat diet (with less than 20 percent of calories derived from fat) may be contraindicated in individuals who suffer both heart disease and depression. Although low-fat diets have demonstrated benefits for some people with heart disease, such diets tend to be seriously deficient in omega-3 fatty acids. Some authorities have proposed that low-fat diets may even contribute to depression because of their low omega-3 content. All too often, low-fat diets are high in carbohydrates. For the 47 million Americans estimated to have metabolic syndrome, a high-carbohydrate diet may magnify heart disease risk. It can also result in most fat intake coming from omega-6 fatty acids, compounds that increase thromboxane A2, a pro-inflammatory and vessel-constrictive agent that contributes to heart disease and may promote the depressive syndrome.

When fish oil is given to people suffering from depression, mood is substantially improved. A small, placebo-controlled trial of 36 patients conducted by Lauren Marangell, M.D., chief of psychopharmacology at the Baylor College of Medicine, demonstrated improved mood in depressed persons following six weeks of treatment with 2 grams per day of DHA. A similar study at the China Medical University in Taiwan compared higher doses of fish oil (9.6 grams per day) with placebo in 28 patients with major depression. Substantial improvement in mood using a standardized rating assessment was experienced only in the group receiving fish oil. In another study, Andrew Stoll, M.D., of Harvard examined 30 patients suffering from difficult-to-treat bipolar disorder (manic depression). Daily consumption of 6.2 grams of EPA and 3.4 grams of DHA resulted in objective improvement in depression scores and longer periods of remission between relapses.

Perhaps the most persuasive clinical evidence documenting the mood benefits of omega-3s was seen in people who already take conventional antidepressant medication. An Israeli study of 20 patients with major depression who were receiving maintenance antidepressant pharmaceutical therapy showed that mood markedly improved after only three weeks of EPA supplementation when compared to placebo. Dr. Malcolm Peet, head of the Omega-3 Mental Health Research Group at the University of Sheffield (England), reported a study of 70 patients on conventional antidepressant therapy. In this trial, dramatic improvement in measures of depression was seen when 1 gram of EPA per day was added to the treatment regimen. Curiously, doses of 2 and 4 grams did not show statistically significant benefits.

Likewise, solid data demonstrate the benefits of omega-3 fatty acids in reducing risk for cardiovascular disease. The Italian GISSI Prevenzione Trial of more than 11,000 participants neatly showed that 850–882 milligrams of EPA and DHA resulted in a 30 percent reduction in death from cardiovascular disease and a 45 percent reduction in sudden cardiac death. These numbers equal or exceed the magnitude of benefits claimed by the cholesterol-reducing statin agents. The large number of participants in the GISSI study makes these observations virtually unassailable. Another study of 360 patients with symptoms of heart attack showed that patients given 1008 milligrams a day of EPA and 720 milligrams a day of DHA suffered 48 percent fewer cardiac deaths and 76 percent fewer sudden cardiac deaths, as well as a 54 percent reduction in dangerous heart rhythms.

Fish oil likely achieves these benefits through a broad spectrum of mechanisms, including increased cell membrane fluidity (affecting signal transduction), suppression of abnormal heart rhythm-generating activity, and marked reductions of triglycerides and the very low-density fraction of lipoproteins that can lead to the formation of dangerous "small" LDL particles and a drop in beneficial HDL. Fish oil also reduces the blood-clotting protein fibrinogen and inhibits platelet aggregation, both of which can prevent blood-clot formation on active, ruptured coronary plaque, which can contribute to a heart attack.

Depression and Heart Disease

In the U.S., prevention of heart disease is an area of huge neglect. Treatment of major depression is likewise an imperfect practice, with less-than-optimal responses to antidepressant medication being an everyday phenomenon. Omega-3 fatty acids may indeed be a missing link that provides substantial benefits in both areas with virtually no downside. While the concomitant treatment of heart disease and depression with fish oil has never been formally examined in a clinical trial, it remains a compelling topic worthy of further examination.

Fish oil is the most concentrated source of the omega-3 fatty acids EPA and DHA. A secondary source is alpha-linolenic acid (ALA), which is found in flaxseed, walnuts, and canola oil. However, only 10 percent of ALA ingested from food is converted into active EPA or DHA; much of it is simply burned for calories. Fish oil thus remains the most potent source of omega-3 fatty acids.

Benefits of Folic Acid and SAMe

Depressed, hostile, or angry people have higher homocysteine levels. If homocysteine leads to coronary plaque growth and heart attack, will folic acid and B vitamins that lower homocysteine improve mood and reduce heart attack?

The data strongly suggest that folic acid supplementation elevates mood, both in people already taking antidepressant medication and in those who are not. Indeed, five clinical trials, though all relatively small (each with fewer than 100 patients), have consistently demonstrated improvements in depression measures when patients are given various doses of folic acid. For instance, in a 1993 study of 96 patients at the University of Parma, Italy, folic acid supplementation yielded improvements in mood similar to those of conventional antidepressants. Another study by Drs. Alec Coppen and John Bailey in Surrey, England, showed that response to prescription fluoxetine (Prozac) was substantially improved by taking as little as 500 micrograms of folic acid a day.

Though few psychiatrists have added folic acid to their arsenal of antidepressant therapeutics, the data suggest that this simple, inexpensive treatment should be a part of every depressed person's panel of therapies. Doses of only 1–5 milligrams would be required, generally along with 25–50 milligrams of vitamin B6. Vitamin B12 should always be taken with folic acid to help guard against a hidden B12 deficiency.

The growing experience with folic acid treatment in people at risk for cardiovascular disease includes three clinical trials suggesting that folic acid reduces the growth of plaque in the carotid arteries (a surrogate for coronary plaque growth) and reduces the likelihood of future heart attack. The Canadian group at the Stroke Prevention and Atherosclerosis Research Centre in Ontario reported an investigation in 101 patients showing that a homocysteine level greater than 14 micromoles per liter (14 μmol/L) identified a group that showed much more rapid growth of carotid plaque. Daily treatment with 2.5 milligrams of folic acid, 25 milligrams of vitamin B6, and 250 micrograms of vitamin B12 eliminated plaque growth. The Dutch group at Vrije Universiteit in Amsterdam has reported extensively on treating high homocysteine levels using folic acid and vitamin B6 in patients with peripheral arterial disease (usually of the leg arteries), which demonstrated the reduction of heart attack, slowed growth of carotid and leg artery plaque, and diminished likelihood of death.

Folic acid supplementation increases levels of the homocysteine metabolite s-adenosyl-L-methionine, or SAMe. Some have speculated that the mood-elevating properties of folic acid may be at least partly due to an increase in endogenous SAMe, since SAMe has been shown in numerous studies to be an effective antidepressant supplement. Since 1973, over 40 clinical trials have demonstrated the effectiveness of SAMe in elevating mood in the depressed, including a total of 537 patients in 13 randomized, double-blind studies. In 18 trials pitting SAMe head to head against the conventional antidepressants imipramine, chlorimipramine, and others, SAMe proved equally effective, and it is essentially without side effects.

SAMe has been available in the U.S. as an over-the-counter supplement since 1997, though it has been available over the counter or by prescription in Europe for over 20 years. SAMe at a dose of 400 milligrams per day yields blood levels in the range believed to induce antidepressant benefits, though some clinicians have noted that doses up to 1600 milligrams daily are required for some individuals. It is interesting to speculate that the combination of folic acid and SAMe might yield even greater benefits and more powerfully improve mood and many of the downstream phenomena leading to coronary disease risk. This remains an area for further research.

Folic acid supplementation, therefore, likely improves mood while lowering homocysteine and thus the risk of heart attack. Along with fish oil and omega-3 fatty acids, folic acid represents another intriguing "missing link" between two disparate diseases with an exciting potential for common treatments.

Depression and Metabolic Syndrome

As the U.S. population gets heavier and heavier, metabolic syndrome becomes increasingly more prevalent. One in every four American adults suffers from this common condition, which represents a combination of lifestyle and genetic factors. Because depressed people are more likely to develop metabolic syndrome, this disorder is another important mediator of the interplay between mood and heart disease.

Most of us have seen someone who, when struck with depression or impaired by other chronic negative emotions, burrows into a lifestyle of physical inactivity and overeating. The resulting weight gain activates all the latent characteristics of the tragically common metabolic syndrome (increased abdominal fat, hypertension, low HDL, resistance to insulin—dubbed "the deadly quartet" by Dr. Norman Kaplan in 1989). This familiar sequence can greatly magnify risk for heart disease.

But can the reverse occur? Can a person become overweight through neglect or indulgence, develop metabolic syndrome, then trigger depression and the cascade of events leading to heart disease? If this flip-flop in the sequence of events were true, then efforts aiming squarely at managing weight and metabolic syndrome should be among our principal health concerns.

A fascinating study conducted by Drs. Katri Raikkonen of the University of Helsinki (Finland) and Lewis Kuller of the University of Pittsburgh attempted to untangle this question. Psychological and metabolic measures were obtained in 425 middle-aged females. Seven and a half years later, these same measures were repeated. Raikkonen and Kuller reported that women with emotional characteristics of anger, depression, and anxiety at initial enrollment were more likely to develop metabolic syndrome. Even more interestingly, women without these psychological traits but with metabolic syndrome at the start were more likely to develop anger, anxiety, and depression by the end of the study. In other words, in this second group, abdominal fat, high blood pressure, low HDL, and insulin resistance—all the features of metabolic syndrome—predicted a future of negative emotions. By either route, the result is a person with the physiological stage set for development of heart disease.

How to Lose Weight Faster

Metabolic syndrome is, in the great majority of cases, a disease of the overweight and obese. If metabolic syndrome leads to depression and other negative emotions that further escalate the risk of heart disease, which is all the more reason to attack metabolic syndrome. Not surprisingly, the most direct, effective way to do so is to lose weight. Weight loss might then be a useful path to reducing the risk of both depression and heart disease. Unfortunately, that is easier said than done.

Carbohydrate-restricted programs, popularized by the Atkins and South Beach diets, in some people are helpful weight-loss tools, though the high-saturated-fat, high-protein, low-fiber approach of the Atkins' "induction phase" makes it unhealthy for a period any longer than several weeks. In the author's experience, people with metabolic syndrome respond in an unhealthy exaggerated manner to these diets, losing weight rapidly. Losses of 10–20 pounds in the first month are not uncommon.

Along with a healthy vegetarian diet, several nutritional supplements can supercharge weight-loss efforts and thereby improve many features of metabolic syndrome. They include:

> *White bean extract.* This supplement blocks intestinal carbohydrate absorption by 66 percent. Taking 1500 milligrams twice a day with meals can lead to 3–7 pounds of weight loss in the first

month of use. Like its prescription counterpart (acarbose), it can cause excess gas, though usually modest. Do not succumb to the temptation to indulge in carbohydrates, since the blocking effect is only partial. You can overcome the effect quite easily, for instance, with a 50-gram carbohydrate load of just two granola bars.

Calcium pyruvate. Doses of 700 milligrams twice a day act as a weight-loss accelerator that is safe and ephedra-free. Calcium pyruvate also has the interesting property of exercise enhancement, making exercise easier and less taxing, and encouraging exercise that is longer and harder with a smoother recovery.

Chromium. This trace mineral provides an insulin-sensitizing benefit along with a modest effect of promoting weight loss. The dose ranges from 600 to 1000 micrograms per day and is best used consistently over a period of several months. Work with your doctor to monitor your blood sugar if you have established diabetes or take medication to lower your blood sugar before you begin taking chromium.

Testosterone. Contrary to popular belief, testosterone supplementation in men is more useful in improving mood than in stoking libido. Feelings of sadness, fatigue, anger, and even severe depression may be associated with declining blood levels of testosterone in men in their 40s and beyond. Testosterone can often result in dramatic improvement in these symptoms. Testosterone not only improves the psychological side of the equation, but also can improve many characteristics of metabolic syndrome through its weight-loss-promoting effects.

Carnitine. This is a supplement that may be equal to testosterone in its ability to improve sexual function, boost low moods, increase energy, and promote weight loss through its effect on fat and glucose metabolism. A dose of 2000 milligrams per day of acetyl-L-carnitine has been found effective in most studies.

DHEA. This is an adrenal hormone whose beneficial effects include its considerable ability to elevate mood, particularly in men and women with lower blood levels of DHEA-sulfate. Among the most persuasive reports is a 1999 study conducted at the National Institute of Mental Health in which 90 milligrams per day of DHEA significantly improved symptoms such as anhedonia (loss of interest), loss of energy, lack of motivation, emotional "numbness," sadness, inability to cope, and worry in men and women aged 45 to 63. DHEA also improves some features of metabolic syndrome by increasing sensitivity to insulin, decreasing constriction of the body's arteries (endothelial function), and reducing plasminogen activator inhibitor-1, a potent blood-clot-promoting protein. The most common dose is 25 milligrams for women aged 45 and older, and 25–50 milligrams for men aged 40 and older.

PGX. This is a highly viscous fiber blend of glucomannan, xanthan, and alginate that limits sugar absorption and the subsequent after-meal insulin spike. This sugar-limiting effect can occur when taking a relatively low dose of 1–3 grams before each meal. A related benefit is a modest reduction in total cholesterol and LDL.

Exercise is another therapeutic tool that simultaneously addresses both metabolic syndrome and risk for heart disease. Exercise is an effective strategy to lose weight, improve insulin sensitivity, and lower levels of stress hormones. Aerobic exercise has the added capacity to improve mood. In fact, 16 weeks of exercise can be as effective as prescription antidepressant medication for depression.

Thyroid Test

Symptoms of depression can be caused by a malfunctioning thyroid gland. When the thyroid is impaired in its ability to regulate metabolism, the self-renewal capacity of the body is greatly reduced. The energetic stagnation that ensues is experienced as depression, fatigue, and listlessness.

Because routine blood tests are not designed to detect serious thyroid malfunctioning, depressive symptoms caused by this disorder are often overlooked and treated as primary depression, thereby missing their real cause.

To self-access thyroid activity, we told participants to place a thermometer under the armpit upon awakening in the morning, before doing anything else and record underarm temperature for seven consecutive days.

For those participants whose body temperature was consistently low, below 98 degrees Fahrenheit, an in-depth thyroid evaluation is recommended in order to obtain appropriate medical treatment for this imbalance.

Endocrine and Immune Regulation and Enhancement

Hormones, neurotransmitters, leukotrienes, cytokines, and

prostaglandins are just some of the microscopic chemical messengers that, under normal circumstances, appropriately initiate, regulate, or terminate many of the biological processes in the body.

These chemicals are constantly being produced, as needed, in response to the challenges and demands of daily life. They are manufactured, stored, activated, sent, received, deciphered, translated into biological changes, and finally recycled or destroyed at every moment of our life.

Levels of these powerful chemicals can become altered as a result of inadequate diet, unhealthy lifestyle, aging coupled with nutritional deficiencies, stressful events, medication, illness, or any other unusual set of circumstances.

When this happens, the whole system of communication in the body can become imbalanced. Overregulation and/or underproduction of compensatory chemicals become the body's strategy, one that often becomes habitual and pathological. It is easy to understand how these imbalances can offset the delicate pattern of chemical brain regulation, precipitating mood changes towards anxiety and/or depression.

For this reason, we felt it was important to obtain a baseline at the beginning of our aforementioned study, whereby the participants' hormonal profile was assessed and recorded. In most cases, we found suboptimal levels of the main hormones such as DHEA, testosterone, progesterone, estrogen, and melatonin, while cortisol levels were abnormally high.

At the end of the three months, without hormonal supplementation or direct regulation by any means other than healthy supportive lifestyle changes, we took a second reading of the participants' hormonal status. We are happy to report that, in 90 percent of the cases, all major levels of hormones had normalized, while cortisol levels had dropped. For participants in their 60s and 70s, these changes were especially remarkable; their hormonal levels had not been that high since their youth.

We took a similar approach when it came to assessing participants' immune status. A baseline of all major immune system markers was taken at the beginning of the study, including measurements of lymphocytes, macrophages, T cells, antigens, and antibodies, among others.

Again, what we found was a consistency of abnormalities ranging from chronic immune suppression to overregulation. As we mentioned above, a very significant improvement in immunity was noted by all participants who had mercury amalgam fillings and then subsequently had them removed. By the end of the study, 90 percent of participants' immune status had normalized with all immune modulators back to normal levels.

From the standpoint of psychoneuroimmunology, our study proves that mental health cannot effectively be addressed as separate from, and independent of, immune processes and overall physical health. In that sense, our study was very complex. We eliminated the dichotomy between body and mind and worked with the organism as a unit, which functions on all levels simultaneously and reflectively.

We feel we have proven that the best and safest treatment modality is established when all symptoms are addressed as pertinent to the totality of who the patient is, as opposed to treating each organ and system as a separate unit that works somewhat independently of the rest of the organism.

We believe that our approach greatly eliminates the need for specialized care of isolated systems or body parts, thereby pointing to the possibility of for a nontoxic, safe and cost-effective approach to mental health and disease prevention in general.

Below we will provide you with protocols to reduce anxiety and depression. Slowly increase dosages, building up to the full protocol recommendations over the course of one month.

NO MORE DEPRESSION OR ANXIETY

You may start by taking a group of suggested supplements (two or three at a time) to see if you have any adverse reactions. The process of elimination for allergy response will be simpler this way.

Protocol for Anxiety

Chromium picolinate, 200 mcg, twice a day

Zinc citrate, 25 mg, twice a day

Selenium, 50 mcg, twice a day

Vitamin B: B1, 50 mg, twice a day; B6, 50 mg, twice a day; B12, 1,000 mcg, once a day; folic acid, 1,000 mcg, once a day; pantothenic acid, 600 mg twice a day; all B vitamins should be taken with food.

Vitamin C with bioflavonoids, 5,000 to 10,000 mg daily

Lead-free calcium citrate, 500 to 1,000 mg daily

EPA/DHA, 1,400 mg of EPA and 1,000 mg of DHA daily

Magnesium citrate, 500 to 1,000 mg daily

5HTP, 100 mg, at bedtime *(Caution: check with your doctor before taking 5HTP if you are on any of the SSRI antidepressants.)*

L-Tyrosine, 1,000 mg, twice a day on an empty stomach *(Caution: do not take L-tyrosine if you are taking an MAO-inhibitor drug.)*

Taurine, 500 mg, twice a day on an empty stomach

EFAs, 3,000 mg daily, plus 200 mg DHA

Melatonin, 5 mg at bedtime

Antioxidant formula blend, take as directed. Commonly

available at vitamin outlets.

Phosphatidylserine and phosphatidycholine complexes, or lechitin granules.

Herbs that have been found helpful in reducing anxiety are: chamomile, valerian, skullcap, passionflower, California poppy, St. John's wort, and linden flower. Use as directed.

Among the more exotic remedies, one that shows great promise is called Adapton. Adapton is a natural alternative to the drugs commonly prescribed for treatment of anxiety disorders. It comes from a species of fish called garum, which is found exclusively off the coast of England.

Adapton's efficacy has been thoroughly tested and confirmed in several studies. It has been found that polypeptides contained in it act as precursors to endorphins and other natural neurotransmitters, plus it contains an omega-3 fatty acid complex that enhances prostaglandins and prostacyclins, which are important chemical mediators of neurological and immune functions. Adapton has an overall beneficial effect on mental outlook and cognitive functions because of its safety and efficacy. It is being prescribed more and more in Europe for treatment of anxiety disorders, such as childhood hyperactivity, attention deficit disorder, and other learning disabilities.

Protocol for Depression

SAMe, 400 mg, 3 to 4 times a day

Phosphatidylserine and choline complexes, 500 mg daily

St. John's wort, 300 mg, twice a day

Gingko Biloba, 400 mg, daily

NO MORE DEPRESSION OR ANXIETY

NADH, 5 to 10 mg, daily

EPA's, 3,000 mg, daily, plus 200 mg DHA

Glutathione, 2,000 mg, daily on an empty stomach

NAC, 1,000 mg, daily on an empty stomach

Micronized creatine, 500 mg, 4 times a day

N-acetylcysteine, 600 mg, once or twice a day

Acetyl-L-carninite, 1,000 mg, twice a day on an empty stomachDl-phenylalanine, 1,000 mg in the morning and 500 mg in the early afternoon *(Caution: do not take dl-phenylalanine if you suffer from panic attacks, diabetes, high blood pressure, or PKU.)*

L-tyrosine, 1,000 mg, 3 times a day on an empty stomach *(Caution: do not take L-tyrosine if you are taking an MAO-inhibitor drug.)*

5 HTP, 100 mg, at bedtime *(Caution: check with your doctor before taking 5HTP if you are on any the SSRI antidepressants.)*

Zinc Citrate, 25 mg, daily

Selenium, 200 mcg, daily

B-complex, 100 mg, daily

Vitamin C with bioflavonoids, 5,000 to 10,000 mg, daily or to bowel tolerance

Vitamin E, 400 IU, daily, and 200 mg gamma-tocopherol

L-phenylalanine, 500 to 1000 mg, in the morning daily

Tyrosine, 500 to 100 mg, daily

Tryptophan, 500 to 1000 mg, once a day on an empty stomach

Antioxidant formula, take as directed on the bottle

Melatonin, 5 mg, at bedtime

Calcium Pyruvate, 2500 mg, twice a day

White Bean Extract, 1500 mg, twice a day

Chromium, 600 to 1000 mcg, daily

Testosterone (for older patients with depression), consult your physician.

Herbs and other remedies that may relieve symptoms of depression: green tea extract, licorice, astragalus, ginseng, ginger, lemon balm, and peppermint teas.

• CHAPTER 7 •

Positive Affirmations

One of the most important steps we can take in caring for ourselves is to keep our mind focused on what is possible. We can and must focus on becoming whole. Otherwise, we will forever be honoring the world of disinformation, distortion, and lies that work against us.

The vast majority of Americans are conscientious, hardworking, and do their level best to try to play by the rules. The trouble is that the rules are manipulated so that we rarely have a chance to survive and thrive with happiness and fulfillment. More often than not, the rules are made by people who lead us to spend money we don't have, to buy things we don't need, and to create debt we can't afford. To manage the resulting stress, they provide us with sublimating activities that cause further victimization—gambling, drugs, alcohol, pornography, compulsive working, and medication. So other people create our problems and then manipulate how we cope with them.

If we're ready to change and fill that emptiness within our lives with meaning, then we have to know that our lives count, that we do not have to accept everyone else's advice or live by their reality. There is a promise to our existence. We honor that purpose by accepting, affirming, and focusing on it and by having positive goals. By doing so, we can regain what is essentially ours.

Positive Affirmations

With this in mind, I have created some affirmations. All I ask is that each day you read a single affirmation and continue to look at it throughout the day. Whenever there is a problem, remind yourself that life is dualistic. For every negative there is a positive, for every crisis a blissful moment, for every breakdown a breakthrough. These affirmations are meant to offer balance in a world that appears to be toxic and out of balance.

This is a true story. During World War II, a group of Jewish women arrived at Auschwitz. They were told to form one line. At the front of this line stood one of Hitler's SS commanders with a baton. If the baton pointed to the right, the woman could work and her life was spared. If the baton pointed to the left, the woman was infirm or too old to work, and she would be killed.

A plain young woman with a withered hand came next in line before the captain. In a small but brave voice, she said, "Good morning, sir." A moment passed before he looked at the woman's useless hand. Another moment. "Yes, it is a good morning," he replied. In a flash, the baton firmly pointed to the right! She was spared because of one life affirming, "Good morning!" Yes, positive energy does yield positive solutions!

A positive frame of mind must be cultivated, much as you would prepare a field to receive seeds. It is unrealistic to expect a positive or receptive mindset to overtake you just because you need it at decision time. Rather, consider the style of President Abraham Lincoln who had prepared himself to make certain life-and-death decisions by determining in advance that the protection of the greatest number of people is required for a wise decision. This was his foundation.

Many deserters were court-martialed during our Civil War, and President Lincoln was often beseeched by relatives of deserters to pardon them. He would accept almost any reason to do so. His positive frame of mind told him that there were enough weeping widows and orphans without creating more by killing the men who had made errors in judgment by running from responsibility. One general in particular who had many deserters in his ranks begged Lincoln to let deserters die on the premise that setting them free would be unfair to the soldiers who stayed and fought. Lincoln vehemently refused because his mind was set to keep bloodshed to a minimum.

However, it must be noted that when a slave trader was sentenced to death, Lincoln staunchly refused to commute his sentence, stating that the man had stolen Africa's people from their homeland and forced them and their children to work here for generations in misery as slaves. A decision to pardon this man was unthinkable to Lincoln because his positive mindset told him that this slave trader had gone out of his way to harm whole families of innocent people for material gain. This was odious to Lincoln because it was in direct opposition to his own philosophy of protecting both the majority and minority whenever possible. Lincoln's decisions were always consistent with his positive foundation. Do you have a positive foundation for your decisions?

I'm now going to share with you a list of affirmations that you can use to get yourself into a positive frame of mind.

1. People who ultimately succeed in life generally have made many more mistakes than other people, but they don't view the mistake as a traumatic endpoint. Mistakes are seen, instead, as launching pads for learning. Edison, the inventor, is a classic example of this technique in which mistakes are welcomed as teachers. The light bulb, now the universal symbol for a brilliant new idea, was perfected only after thousands of errors led Edison patiently to its discovery. Never give up!

2. I have never seen a situation that was so bad that

Positive Affirmations

being positive couldn't improve. Positive energy yields solutions; negative energy never does.

3. That which creates comfort can create complacency. Complacency stops the growth process. The mother bear hibernates comfortably all winter in the grip of passivity, but she does not grow. To grow, she must awaken and abandon the security of her cave to find food. She must return to the world and the needs of her cubs. So must you. Your world family needs you.

4. When you live in the moment, life is simple.

5. Do you volunteer to be a victim? Does this bring you redemption, love, sympathy, or ultimately rejection when people get tired of hearing about your troubles? Can you see the cycle of self-hatred here? Has your desperate need for attention led you to seek out something to complain about? Stop blaming. Start growing.

6. Has your stuff become more important than your life? Do you lose sleep worrying about your car? Has the computer replaced your best friend? Have you had your cell phone surgically attached to your ear? If so, it's time to pare down to the bare essentials of life. Go camping! Leave that TV at home! Lighten your load. Downsize to make life simple again.

7. Don't allow someone else to control how you feel. No one should have the power to make you miserable unless you secretly welcome the misery. We like to star in our own dramas.

8. Your best education comes through life—especially through making mistakes, being humiliated, feeling stupid, and being embarrassed. Now don't run after

these. They find all of us for own benefit and so we don't take ourselves too seriously and go around hurting people with our arrogance and inflated egos.

9. Much of what we think, feel, and do every day is based on preconceived notions. When you cling to fixed expectations, you are bound to be disappointed and to become upset frequently. For example, if you believe that everyone you know should greet you with a smile, you're setting yourself up for what you perceive as insults, which leads to feelings of fear, grief, and anger afterwards. This is self-sabotage. Live more in the moment.

10. I thought that if I could do enough, I'd be enough. I did more than enough, but I don't feel like I am enough. I am sacred. I do not have to do anything; by just being alive, I am enough.

11. Do you fear change? Why? What happens when you are forced to change? What happens when you choose something? You have to be responsible for the choice you make. Actually, greed also partly explains our fear to commit to a choice. Think of all the options we lose when we favor just one.

12. Be responsible for your actions. Criminals take all the credit when they get away with something, but they never want to take the blame when they get caught. "Incorrigibles" are often raised in homes or on the streets where mischief is rewarded subtly at an early age. The message is, "Get away with as much as you can." Disgrace is getting nailed for the crime. The crime itself is winked at in this mindset. Are you winking at crime? Flirting with inflicting suffering on others is a dangerous game. Taking responsibility

Positive Affirmations

for your actions is more a step towards growth.

13. Don't tackle a crisis by addressing the symptoms. Deal with the causes.

14. Do your actions and your lifestyle reflect your inner beliefs?

15. How can you get involved and help people without becoming a victim in the process? It's about sacrifice! I must accept there are sacrifices that will occur in all service, but they needn't be fatal.

16. Are you a person who waits for things to change, or do you make things change? How little comes to you if you are waiting? Everything is there; find it. There is little probability that things are going to interfere with your life to make it better. You are fully responsible for that. So stop waiting for things to change. Change them!

17. You're not going to change society by changing yourself to be accepted by society. Your unique contribution, which may be to rebel and correct, will be lost forever if you take the more comfortable road and adapt. You will have lost your mission!

18. Make your most important decisions in a positive frame of mind.

19. Life is a series of passages through which all people assist us.

20. We remember the best experiences of our lives, and we look around to see if it will happen again, and it rarely does. Can you look at each experience with fresh eyes?

21. What we deny, we cannot change.

22. We should only have to hear something that is important once.

23. The more prepared you are, the more open you are, the more opportunities will come to you.

24. When you have used love to meet a challenge and to overcome an obstacle, you are connected to your bliss.

25. The present allows you to have a non-conflict moment. When you are present, you'll make no excuses for the past. You will no longer use the negative experiences of yesterday to deny the completeness of today.

26. If you need someone to love you, it means you need someone else to validate you. You are depending on another for your self-esteem.

27. People confuse what they do with who they are. You are more relevant than your work or possessions.

28. None of us has complete control over what happens to us. Live as if today counts.

29. We must be open to ideas that challenge our own beliefs in order to grow.

30. If your relationship does not honor your needs, then reevaluate why you're still trying to make it work. What are you trying to prove?

31. Not to do something is also a conscious choice.

32. Wisdom transcends knowledge.

33. When we receive praise and respect from others, we tell ourselves that others like us. This is what

happens when we are externally driven by what we create as our reality. We have to ask ourselves if we would like ourselves without the recognition of others.

34. We tend to base too much in our lives on external realities.

35. We should ask ourselves what we have sacrificed spiritually in order to have our standard of living.

36. We cling to permanent religious beliefs, permanent social beliefs, and permanent political beliefs.

37. Think of the things in our lives you want to keep forever. You may want your kids to be kids forever, and then one day everyone grows up. Much of our anxiety comes from the anger we feel because we've lost the present moment by focusing our energy on the past or on the future. We're so preoccupied with gaining something from the future that we lose what we have in the present. By looking forward, how can you know where you are? Live in this moment.

38. All we have is this moment, nothing else.

39. Most people want more than the moment. We want to recapture the moment, which we cannot do. To paraphrase a Greek philosopher, "You can never step twice into the same river." That is because no two moments in a river's history are the same. It may take the same course, but every drop of water flowing by is different. What we have to appreciate is that every moment in every day of our lives is different. No two kisses are the same. No two meals are the same. Your joy comes from just being in this unique moment.

40. How can I honor my inner self if my whole world is based on my external self? The truth is there is no self.

41. Everything you do is a choice.

42. The ego binds the intellect.

43. It is only the internal process that allows us to understand the external in which we live.

44. A "joy journal" lets us know something we thought or did or shared with someone was so important to us that we found utter joy in it. It's important to see how much joy we are allowing into our lives.

45. Look for a person who is healthy and happy, and then ask them for some guidance.

46. There is a difference between your conditioned wants and your essential needs. Only allow into your life what is really missing.

47. The only thing that is uniquely yours is your time.

48. Listen to someone without becoming the critic. Listen neutrally and learn.

49. We like to believe that all people are the same. No one is the same as anyone else. Everyone is different. We don't honor our differences. We like to collectivize people.

    It is a fascinating fact that no two human bodies are identical. Each human heart is shaped just a bit differently. The pattern of the arteries varies; the contours of the livers are not the same; the kidneys are never suspended in quite the same way.

Positive Affirmations

Immunity also varies from person to person. Two people may walk down the same street and get stung on their left thumbs by two bees. The first person barely gets a welt out of it and in two hours, the other person is dead.

The fact that each human body is unique means that each of us occupies a special position on this earth. No one can replace another.

50. Time is the same for everyone. It's what we do with it that makes a difference.

51. Accept everyone as being beautiful until they show that he or she is not.

52. Trust that everything you need to express and everything you need to communicate is already in place. All you have to do is get out of the way and allow it to express itself.

53. Honor and enjoy what you have! Appreciation is the secret of true success—the kind you cannot lose.

54. In our world, we have learned to gain at someone else's loss. Is that humane?

55. How many times in your life have you set a goal that no one else could achieve? Be realistic. Set goals slightly above your comfort zone to create discomfort in order to grow.

56. We like to think that we are something that we are not in order to compensate for our fear of feeling inadequate as we are.

57. No matter where you run, you take your negative thoughts with you. Try traveling light instead.

Surrender your mind to the moment. Let the moment win your full attention! The sun is rising to distract you from your negative thoughts! The whole universe is charged with this compassionate mission to rescue you from your busy mind!

58. Don't make success more important than happiness. Happiness is a real emotion, but success can be an illusion.

59. Sometimes we work so hard to be someplace else; we don't pay attention to the present. This is how we lose the appreciation of beauty in our lives!

60. Surrender your ego! Violence and the need for rigid control will die with it!

61. When you realize that other people do have a right to life, then they become sacred to you. We all like to be loved, honored, and recognized.

62. Dynamic people live by challenges. It's only through challenge that you're forced to use your strengths. Challenge brings out the best in us. So why don't you bring challenge into your everyday life? Live by challenge!

63. Your thoughts create fear. How you've been conditioned determines how you are going to bring your thoughts together.

64. You can only feel good when you think of something that allows you to feel good; you can only feel bad when you think of something that allows you to feel bad.

65. What science doesn't understand, it doesn't accept.

Positive Affirmations

66. Choices you make often have nothing to do with what is going on now.//
67. How many times do we become what we fear?
68. There's no perfection; it takes 1,000 honest mistakes to master life.
69. If you stay in the moment, you're processing wellness.
70. Energy is the basis of all life.
71. Procrastination is an excuse not to go forward.
72. We don't like to make changes because we don't like how it feels when we're going to lose something.
73. We have too many things in our lives that are superficial and not essential.
74. People who are happy don't have to spend their lives sublimating and escaping to all kinds of other activities.
75. In the presence of happiness, everything else becomes less significant.
76. When people mistrust other people, usually it's because they don't trust themselves.
77. Growth is easy when you have a silent mind.
78. What empowers you is the respect you give yourself.
79. We have to disconnect from the nonessential to reconnect with what is essential.
80. Do not be distracted by others' goals.
81. We have a constant need to have a certain image. Why?

82. We have become an achievement-oriented society. In the past 30 years, there were over 5 million baby-boomer millionaires. Now there are almost 1 million baby-boomer millionaires each year. Their whole emphasis is upon the idea that the more I have and the more I own and the more I accomplish and the more I achieve, the more someone is going to respect who I am.

83. Our impermanence scares us.

84. We want everything good to last. We hate loss. This is one source of suffering.

85. You cannot do anything until you engage energy. Engaging the energy precipitates the crisis that leads to change, which brings health.

86. My life works because I make it work. If my life doesn't work, it's because I allow it not to work. If I go into a championship race, I cannot expect to win if I have not trained as a champion.

87. Any time you act opposite to how you naturally are, you won't be fulfilled in what in whatever it is you are doing. That's why dynamic people should not work for anyone else. Be who you are!

88. Emotions cannot occur unless there is a thought. You create a thought, your thought has an image, the image creates an emotion, and the emotion creates your reaction.

89. We don't know how to rest. When was the last time you spent a day without a cell phone, radio, the Internet, TV, or talking?

90. Strip us all naked and take away our titles and we're

Positive Affirmations

just human beings. It doesn't matter if we're Jewish, Catholic, black, white, rich, or poor. Cut us and we all bleed the same red blood.

91. We are not so uniquely different from one another; we pretend to be because that's how we get our image.

92. Go in and embrace your biggest fears. You'll see that fear is mainly an illusion.

93. Think of how many passages you've been through in life. You have the right to change course; you can go on a hundred paths if you wish.

94. Most of the things we fear losing are imprisoning us.

95. What is the root of envy and jealousy? Is it real or perceived? It is pain from the past, such as sibling rivalry, insidiously triggering pain in the present where there is no real cause for pain.

96. If you're my friend, I don't care what you are. I just care that you're a good person. I like you as a friend. If you're in trouble, I'm going to help you. If you fall down, I'm going to kneel down and pick you up. That's what friends do.

97. Here's the rule: anyone who's going to gossip to you is going to gossip about you.

98. I'd rather live in a one-room apartment and have unconditional time with the one I love than live in a mansion with a stranger.

99. You pay the price for success. The smart person says no to opportunity once in a while.

100. Do you dissipate energy by doing too much and not doing anything completely?

101. What you want to change may not really need to change. To change what you need to change takes honesty and the courage to sacrifice old habits.

102. Procrastination restricts energy. Action liberates it. Either way you are going to feel energy; one's depleted, one's enhanced. Which do you want?

103. We are on automatic selection instead of making choices in the present.

104. It's worth going through temporary discomfort to get a health benefit.

105. When we look in the mirror, we should look at what we ideally want to see. Every time you look in the mirror you should see the ideal body. If all you see is what you have, then you're going to be limited by the vision of what you have as all that you're capable of being.

106. "Hard" to me is holding onto something that doesn't work, despite having given it a fair chance.

107. Look for the reasons why you should do what you want to do. Encourage yourself to take action.

108. Don't look for someone or something to change your life. Rescue yourself! Read Emerson's essay on "Self-Reliance."

109. How can you trust someone who is egocentric, powerful, and self-centered? You need to have confidence in yourself, and find understanding and balance in life to achieve independence. No one's power should exceed your own. You need to be the strongest person in your life.

Positive Affirmations

110. We inevitably compare friends, lovers, achievements, and experiences, but this dishonors our present circumstances. Accept where you are in the present moment and be happy.

111. Visualize your achievements and focus your energy and passion, then move fearlessly toward accomplishing your goals. Forget the expectations of others and your conditioning. Take chances; don't be afraid of others' opinions of you. Be creative and work towards your life.

112. What we give up is important. We should relinquish fears and limitations to gain new understanding and possibilities of feelings, creativity, etc.

113. Do this daily: Don't compromise the essential self and negate that value. Appreciate self in spite of others. Often, you are the only person who will stand up for you. Be who you are. Don't be afraid of taking a chance to be you by staying "safe" and predictable.

114. Every painful experience strengthens you for the next one.

115. Remember: growth may threaten others; they don't want a challenge to negate themselves. So, don't look to others for self-validation. You have to validate yourself.

116. Desire and motivation are keys to accomplishment. You can find ways to use the inherent crises in life as tools to help you grow. If you think you have insurmountable problems and you need inspiration, read *The Story of My Life* by Helen Keller.

117. Eliminate the words "but" and "can't" from your vocabulary and from your life. They will limit and

restrict you. Without those words, you can accomplish your goals. Prepare to succeed. Don't allow yourself or others to restrict your progress.

118. Don't impose artificial limits on yourself; discard them.

119. What I want from you in a relationship is quality companionship that is honest and open and vivacious, and dynamic conversation with commitment to an ideal or standard of sharing that never abuses trust.

120. Are you ready for what you want?

121. We cannot do something negative and harmful and then seek a spiritual answer. Does the word "hypocrite" spring readily to mind? How about "sneaky"?

122. You have to do what you want to connect to.

123. No more negative talk.

124. See the ideal that you want to be.

125. Do not mirror anything that makes you feel bad about who you are.

126. You can only care about what you are connected to.

127. When you make the right connection, you do not have to prove anything.

128. Until you can rebel against your complacency, you cannot change.

129. What value did this day have?

130. When you stop fearing change, anything is possible.

Positive Affirmations

131. Stop living at the lowest end of everything.

132. Think of all the (lawful) things you have not done because your beliefs would not allow it.

133. Withdraw from deception and reconnect with honesty.

134. We rarely listen to the person with whom we are in conflict.

135. How can you expand your consciousness if you do not first expand your ideals?

136. Seek what has not yet been discovered; be willing to search for answers that have not yet been found.

137. How many times have you resisted a challenge because you do not like the idea of being challenged?

138. Identify where you drifted away from your own dreams.

139. Recognize opportunity; don't recognize failure. If someone says, "It's a failure," you should see it as an opportunity. Put this thought into your program for growth.

140. Lighten up, loosen up, unwind, and put down your defense mechanisms.

141. If you can't be healthy and whole as an autonomous single, then you'll never be happy in a relationship.

142. Start realizing that what you fear and avoid is what you are. By welcoming new activities, keeping your focus, and taking one more step every day, at the end of the week, your old self recedes, and your new self appears. Get beyond procrastination because in a

year from now if you continue to procrastinate, your health will be worse, your mind will be down, your spirit will be broken and life will be beyond you!

143. Take a look at your life. Is it integrated? It must be integrated to be in harmony. Anything that creates conflict creates crisis.

144. Closure is so important in life.

145. Think integral!

146. Be like a bird. A bird never contemplates its own death while it's flying.

147. Think of a career that would allow you to do the things that fit your life energy.

148. Network your life energy. Partner with someone who will complement your life energy.

149. When you discover what you should be doing, it will be a revelation. You will not have to work at it or sell yourself into it. If you have to sell yourself into it, it's not for you.

150. You can only have happy positive feelings if you have happy positive thoughts.

151. Know that your attitude will change your life!

152. There is nothing more damaging than a mind that is overly critical of itself and/or of others.

153. Stop overreaching to everything. Use reason.

154. I have to change me, not the circumstances of my life.

155. Health simplifies life.

Positive Affirmations

156. We must choose to change or we will be forced by some outside force to change. We must be in control of the change.

157. Do not allow your pain or disease to become more important than you are.

158. The only people you are able to help are those with you in that moment.

159. My life should have quality and meaning beyond my work.

160. Do you blame or complain, or change?

161. We overvalue our possessions and undervalue ourselves.

162. What is so important in the goal that you lose everything in achieving it?

163. Nothing in life is predictable except complacency.

164. You do not need anyone else to make you complete or whole.

165. Knowledge is both the most important quality to gain and to surrender. Don't always look for new knowledge but rather seek a new meaning.

166. Most people live predictable lives. There is no potential in predictable patterns. The world is constantly changing; so should we. The only time people change is when they are in crisis or when there are no other options, e.g., pioneers. To accomplish changes:

    a. People should find a good support system from people who have excelled in their accomplishments.

b. Be in the moment; that's when you are most able to change. The moment cannot exist if you control it. We are never free until we disengage the mind.
   c. Changes should be radical, not small.
   d. Life should be constantly changing.
   e. Nothing ever changes unless we confront it.
   f. Look for the hero.

167. We are born perfect, and we spend the rest of our lives denying it.

168. If you don't try to create an image to please other people, then you are able to create a life that's based upon what you really want.

169. When we are rigid in our comforts and standards, then we become inflexible.

170. You must look beyond your limitations to be able to transcend a problem. Do not criticize yourself; it's a growth process. Failure doesn't exist if you are being yourself.

171. You will always get confronted with what you fear more than what you have mastered. Fear should not dictate what you will or will not do.

172. Winning is not important, it's merely a by-product of attaining excellence.

173. Euphoria and bliss can only occur when the conscious mind has been suspended, surrendered to the moment. It happens to us when we interact with nature and animals.

174. Writing down what's meaningful in your life and

Positive Affirmations

picturing where you want to be is an important part of the changing process.

175. The more time you spend with someone, the more time you see that part of him that's hidden. We need to have more time to ourselves, rather than spend every minute with another person. Allow more personal space.

176. How many times have you made decisions based on your need to control everything, and based on your discomfort when you can't control things?

177. What we cannot control, we generally destroy. We marginalize.

178. And needing to control a relationship, an environment, a people, a moment, means that there's not a free flow of energy.

179. What do we do to control the uncertainty of our lives? We try to make things certain. And how do we make things certain? We try to make them permanent.

180. Love is not something someone can give you. Love is something you feel, and you express it by how you live.

181. It's only when you're vulnerable that you grow, because you are giving yourself the freedom to make errors. And you better learn to be happy with the mistakes you make, because if you are angry at the mistakes you make, then you create a self-loathing.

182. Only the quiet mind can heal.

183. And stop trying to figure everything out. Life was

never meant to be figured out, it was meant to be lived. There is a big difference.

184. You can either adapt to a situation or transcend boundaries.

185. Stress is not an external happening. Change your reaction and you change the outcome of the stress.

186. Being skilled and successful are not enough after all.

187. Every day, include small, optimistic, joyful events. Break your daily ritual. That's one way we can change how we deal with stress because we're now going to make every day a ritual of happiness. Play with a pet, grow flowers, listen to music, prepare a dish to eat, or write to a friend.

188. How is fear used to control us?

189. We look for the medications that keep us comfortable in our suffering.

190. What would you do if fear was not an option?

191. If you need someone to love you and to validate you, then it's not love you're seeking, it's validation. Don't call it love. It's need.

192. Are you going to waste a lot of your time trying to be complete with someone else?

193. What you do not address and what you do not change and what you do not reconcile in yourself, you take into a relationship, and now all you have is the incompleteness of two needy people coming together, even if your needs are similar. And all you still have is the insecurity and the stress of knowing you're still incomplete, but in that relationship you are going to

try to disguise your incompleteness for fear of having the other person recognize it.

194. We may bond with someone superficially, and we wrap it in emotion and sexual obligation and all forms of commitments, but the first time that is stressed, it breaks.

195. Challenge your relationship, challenge anything in your life you feel is inessential, and see whether or not you withstand the challenge and are stronger because of it.

196. I'm suggesting to look at your truths one at a time. Analyze them and say, "Is this truth a universal one?" Could his apply to everyone? And if it can't, then surrender it.

197. Do you only accept information that supports your viewpoints? Do you ignore everything else? That is how we manifest disease—not honoring who we really are. And not honoring our core values.

198. Adaptation keeps you in the circle of the known. Transformation transcends the known. Transformation is where the healing is— it is not in adaptation.

199. Choose a project that forces you to test your beliefs.

200. When we no longer carry blame and shame, then self-love evolves. Stop criticizing.

201. When we are accountable on a daily basis for our basic and essential needs, then we prevent conflict.

202. How do you validate what is accurate or distorted? How do you know that what you believe is real?

203. Are you motivated by outside pressures to do something? Why do you do what you do? And who or what causes you to do it?

204. Do you function from conscious choice (meaning making proper decisions about your life) or fear (by default)?

205. Education provides tools and rituals but no spiritual context in which to use them.

206. Fear equals anger. Anger equals unhappiness. Unhappiness equals resentment. Resentment equals greed. Greed equals obsession and the need to dominate. And that all equals violence. So if you want to look at the extension of violence, go back to what precedes it. Don't just look at the final act. Look at everything that came before it. It's all part of it.

207. We either fear doing something or remember what we did and didn't like. So you shouldn't be caught in the past and you shouldn't be projecting your fear into the future. Life is the moment. Wisdom transcends knowledge in the capacity to function and make proper choices.

208. How often do you remind yourself of past mistakes?

209. Change the word mistake into experience.

210. I will continue to learn because I'm not afraid to make mistakes.

211. Do you hide from conflict? Do you try to please others?

212. Which rules do you use to prevent risks?

213. No risks, no rewards. Little risks, little rewards. Big

risks, big rewards.

214. Only when you believe you are enough to be complete in your own life without anyone else's input about what you should, what you should think, and what you should be, are you going to realize that you can start all over again and recreate your values.

215. Every person has the capacity to change.

216. Start a day only with positive thoughts: I am going to honor my body, mind, heart, and spirit.

217. People confuse the idea of being in love with need. The whole idea of a relationship is to enhance each other's life, rather than to be dependent on each other.

218. If you can't change something, change the perception of it, so it won't control you.

219. Rediscover your inner child. Every day, bring up the qualities of childhood: innocence, honesty, curiosity, wonderment, creativity, adaptability, forgiveness, happiness, energy, eagerness to learn, spontaneity, trusting others, lack of inhibition, dreaming the impossible, heroism, no self-condemnation, optimism, playfulness, resourcefulness, and love.

220. Love yourself unconditionally!

221. What establishes the limits to what you can or are willing to achieve?

222. Ah! Being skilled and successful are not enough after all. List how've you've used your skills to create problems for yourself and others.

223. What would you do if fear was not an option?

224. When we no longer carry blame, shame, and self-criticism, then self-love evolves.

225. What do you distort about your view of yourself? What don't you see accurately?

226. How do you validate what is accurate or distorted?

227. What is the motivation for what you do?

228. What in our lives is too complicated? What is very simple?

229. What role do dealings, schedules, goals, and play have in our days?

230. Do we have excellent achievements but not so excellent connections to our real needs?

231. Stop doing anything that is not worth doing.

232. Do you obsess on a single issue, or do you bring variety to your thoughts?

233. Images are not reality.

234. What if most of your fears and shortcomings were just wrong projections?

235. You have the right to design your own life.

236. The eye that sees or the ear that hears is first connected to the past self. If anything is remembered as threatening we may automatically reject it, or if something is remembered as acceptable, we are inclined to embrace it.

237. Our fears are disabling. They prevent us from ever testing them. Are they real?

Positive Affirmations

238. If you believe that you are a failure because you didn't do it right, then everyone's expectation of you, including your own, will be lowered.

239. We wait for that special something to appear and ignite our interest, to inspire us into action. We whine and complain like spoiled children for something to occur, while we ourselves are unwilling to do anything and actually make it happen.

240. Don't attack or avoid that which could change your reality. *Don't let fear embalm your beliefs!*

241. When we listen non-judgmentally, we hear everything.

242. In order to believe you can be free or do anything, first you must believe in your completeness.

243. The birth of any new idea, self-actualized, means the death of what it is replacing.

244. Life is in constant change. Do we fear the process of that change?

245. Can you expand your consciousness without first expanding your ideas and values?

246. You resist whatever challenges you.

247. To achieve a meaningful and purposeful goal, we should love it.

248. How often do you say exactly what you feel, believe, expect, and need?

249. To what do you completely commit yourself?

250. Which questions and issues do we avoid or allow others to answer for us?

251. As we age, what triggers our need for purpose?

252. Don't ask *how*—affirm *when* you will engage in a transformational process.

253. Are our goals more important than our lives?

254. What boundaries have we accepted from others as if they were our own?

255. Do we control through reward, punishment, or unconditional encouragement?

256. When we strive for constant security and happiness, we create stress as each circumstance evolves.

257. Don't accept your imperfection as limitation.

258. Did you choose change or were you forced into it?

259. How do you validate your life? For whom do you do it? We are merely an extension of the common value system of others.

260. What if we choose to reinterpret all of our "realities"? What would change?

261. How does conflict ensue from the need to be right?

262. If you were to step back and look at every part of your life, which part represents the real you? Which parts are authentic? What do your choices reveal about you?

263. Every belief will cause corresponding behavior; examine your behavior if you want to know what you think!

264. Are repetitive thoughts or feelings about any limitation only reinforcing them?

Positive Affirmations

265. If you crave something that you don't have and may never have, how does that influence the present moment?

266. What will loss and change create?

267. We are frequently disappointed because we are not conscious of the moment; instead, we retreat to the past or project the future. We just want to be somewhere else, feeling or experiencing something else.

268. When you master the everyday habit of just being nice, in time it just becomes effortless.

269. Don't expect or even ask for thanks. Do good because you are good.

270. What happens when we compare ourselves to others or allow others to compare themselves to us?

271. Think of the little kindnesses you've received. What do you remember about those moments?

272. Focus on the deep pain that you have survived and replace it with kindness.

273. How can we escape the circle of being a victim?

274. Do you risk being unhappy by growing and changing yourself?

275. What situations have you placed yourself in that you have regretted, but did not have the courage to change?

276. Is challenging yourself to be in motion a dare to surrender each moment?

277. Does the birth of any new idea, self-actualized, mean

the death of what it is replacing? Is life in constant change? Do we fear the process of that change?

278. Which questions and answers do we avoid or let others answer for us?

279. What opportunities does adversity offer?

280. What do you do that really matters?

281. Change is a matter of letting go. What have you let go of?

282. What in our lives is complete?

283. The more you need others, the less you validate yourself. Describe which of your relationships are/were based on "need" that affected your perceptions of your worth and validity.

284. When you transcend, you automatically grow. What have you transcended up to this point? (Include fears, bad habits, destructive jobs, and destructive relationships, toxic foods, procrastination, excuses, etc.)

285. What do you overdo?

286. What do we do to prevent ourselves from being loved?

287. What do we do to prevent ourselves from being financially secure?

288. List five things you do to prevent yourself from being happy.

289. What illusions of security are you still clinging to? (Include food, relationships, money, career, pension, and daily habits.)

Positive Affirmations

290. Compose forgiveness letters:

    a. Make a list of all people, past and present, who hurt you or prevented you from reaching your potential.

    b. Write letters to them sharing what they did and how it affected you in detail. Don't worry about penmanship, grammar, or choice of words. At the end of each letter write the phrase, "and I forgive you." And sign your name.

    c. Write a letter to yourself, outlining anything you have engaged in that is self-denigrating, self-destructive, or counterproductive in your life. Also include anything you may have done to hurt anyone else. And forgive yourself.

    d. Burn the letters.

291. All of our happiness is based in the pursuit and acceptance of the pleasures of our possessions—from people to places to jobs.

292. When you look back on your life, it's all those special and ordinary moments that matter.

293. Our crises always tell us something.

294. Every crisis has its resolution built in and every resolution can prevent its crisis.

295. If we start taking off all the masks everyone wears and all that pretense, we are just left with the same little boys and girls in the playground of life.

296. All the time, I see people who are physically sick because they are sick of their lives.

297. When we feel discomfort, what is our first response? What we should say is, "I don't feel good right now, but I'm going to learn from this. This is an experience that I'm not going to want to repeat and the only way I'm not going to repeat it is to learn from it."

298. Whenever problems are not honestly addressed, they are going to appear in other forms. So what does that tell us about addressing problems? Go right up to it, and look it right in the eye no matter what it is.

299. Think of what happens when you're no longer afraid of losing anything. What have you got in its place? Everything. You've got freedom!

300. How many people end up wasting a lot of their time trying to go through life achieving things to prove they are okay?

301. It's not important who does not accept you; it's only important who does.

302. Anything you've done that does not bring you inner peace and satisfaction has been a test of your time. You've only got so much time and when it's gone, that's it. There's a day you wake up and you're no longer able to do everything that you could have. The opportunity is not always going to be there, and we don't want to live with the anxiety of having missed life because we were too afraid to break the control that other have had. The day that has meaning is the day that you retake your life.

303. It's very easy to keep doing forever what you have been used to doing and can do well—that's protectionism. But what about going into areas you don't know anything about and starting from

Positive Affirmations

scratch? That means you've got to study, you have to learn. You have to be a constant learner about life, which means you have to learn other people's perspectives and other people's ideas and you have to see where balance and imbalance exist.

304. Needing to win shows that without winning, you feel you are a failure. Always look to see what is motivating you. If you need something, then it means without it you're not going to feel good. Winning is fine as long as you can cooperate, not just compete.

305. People who are insecure need to win or never try.

306. What would you do in your life if you weren't afraid of failure?

307. Look at problems as a way of transforming yourself.

308. When you need reward and acknowledgment, you are forced to comply.

309. With every single thing that I do, I must value my consciousness, because my consciousness is the deeper, more insightful, and always honest self. I was born with it. I didn't create it. It was given to me. It's a gift. We are all given a perfect consciousness. Our consciousness allows us to make the decision to do something that is ethical and right.

310. Something great happens when conscious people start sharing energy. You create a fusion of consciousness and now you have power.

311. Remember, every cell in the body, if it's infected by a virus or bacterium, it is affected by something greater. The real healing of the cell is the consciousness of the cell. No cell exists without a consciousness—no

cell. Tap that consciousness and you tap your healing power.

312. When you give 100 percent, and it wasn't enough, what does that tell you? You are giving it to the wrong goal. It shows that the people you are giving it to do not respect what you have given them.

313. How do we match our real needs? The inner voice lets us know. Break the pattern of behavior. If the pattern of behavior has led to the disease in the environment, then change the environment and the pattern.

314. Trust should be earned by our actions, not just by our words.

315. The only people to have in your life are people that can be consistent in honesty, decency, trust, and kindness.

316. If you don't have the confidence of the inner self, then you are always going to be looking for feedback and acceptance from others.

317. Think of all of the things that would change if you had love in your heart all of the time!

318. No matter what, there's still love here, and as long as there's love, there's the capacity to heal.

319. The trouble is that we've never even learned how to use our minds. Using the mind is not worrying about things—that's never achieved anything. Using the mind is not over-concentration; it's not obsessive thoughts or obsessive behavior. It relaxing and surrendering to that which is most natural. And what's most natural is the curiosity, the wonderment, the joy, the grace, the loving, the innocence, and the

Positive Affirmations

honesty to explore life.

320. People who are engaged in life don't think about it.

321. When the world gets to where we don't want to deal with it, we retreat into denial.

322. Eighty percent of a person's given day is engaged in fantasy or escapism. This means that 80 percent of the time is devoted to something else instead of constructively living your life. Imagine what would happen if you started to turn that fantasy into reality.

323. If you don't have a commitment to your higher self, then you commit yourself to the lower self. And the lower self is indulgence and distraction.

324. Spirit allows you to face the crisis and still be okay.

325. Change comes when we seek truth above all superficiality.

326. So much energy is put into deception and into keeping the deception going.

327. That which honors life is true.

328. How are we ever going to communicate with meaning if we are always communicating with partial deception?

329. Make the right choice—the right choice is the honest choice—not the short-term satisfaction.

330. Stress is not an external happening rather it is a reaction to what we can't control. Change your reaction and you can prevent stress.

331. General George S. Patton said, "If everybody is thinking alike, then somebody isn't thinking."

332. Your conditioning and your fear of losing control of a situation will keep you using one tool over and over again, even when that tool hasn't helped you.

333. Spiritual truth gives you courage.

334. "The man who goes alone can start today; but he who travels with another must wait till the other is ready." – Henry David Thoreau, 1854

335. Stress comes when you force something to work.

336. The mind that creates the problem cannot be the mind that solves the problem; you need a new mind, or you'll be answering new questions with the old answers you were spoon-fed.

337. To look at the extension of violence, go back to what precedes it. Don't just look at the final act, look at all that came before it. That's all part of it.

338. All of life is transparent!

339. Connect with that which is blissful, and you will no longer do anything destructive!

• CHAPTER 8 •

Mood-Altering Recipes

When people are either anxious or depressed, they may overeat or lose their appetite altogether. Rarely do they eat what is good for them. When they do eat, people generally go for junk foods or comfort foods. That's when the sugar binging and the chocolate and the pizzas become a form of medication.

For a healthy recovery, we must realize that the mind is nourished by positive thoughts, the brain by positive nutrients. We now know that such nutrients as phosphytitleserine, acetyl-L-carnitine, gingko biloba, L-carnitine, choline, B12 are all important for proper brain function, as is glutathione and essential fatty acids.

When our diet does not contain the nutrients that are the basic building blocks of a healthy body, then we shouldn't be surprised when, at the end of the day, we do not feel better. We are overfed and undernourished, consuming too many calories from protein and fat and not enough nutrients. We are starving for living foods that have a vital life force, foods that cleanse, detoxify, and flood the body with healing phytonutrients.

This chapter is designed to give you the basic tools—juices and solid foods that are tasty, delicious, easy to prepare, and inexpensive. These foods help the body rebalance its chemistry. Frequently that, in and of itself, is enough to

NO MORE DEPRESSION OR ANXIETY

give many people a sense of well-being. Follow this diet and you are going to lose weight, cleanse, naturally chelate toxic metals, and stop body pollution. Eliminating toxic foods is the first step. Rebuilding the body with good foods is the second.

Following a good diet is not always easy to do and may take conscious effort. I travel throughout the United States when I am on tour. Recently I was in Denver, Detroit, Pittsburgh, Washington, D.C., Atlanta, and Fort Myers, all in five days. Wherever I traveled, the hotel restaurant food was not what I would consider healthy. The average American, whether at home or on the road, is consuming an enormous amount of unhealthy foods.

The recipes in this chapter are designed to correct that by getting you on the road to healthy eating. You can also go to your library and get *The Joy of Juicing Cookbook*, *The International Vegetarian Gourmet Cookbook*, *The New Vegetarian Cookbook*, and *Vegetarian Cooking for Good Health*. Feel free to substitute items, where necessary. In my early cookbooks, I included dairy, assuming that organic milk would be fine. Today I would replace that with rice milk or soymilk. Historically, I used organic flour. Today I exclude that and instead use spelt, amaranth, quinoa, millet, oat, or brown rice.

I find that people on a wheat-free, dairy-free, sugar-free, caffeine-free diet have more energy and less weight; they begin to feel better and look better. Sometimes that's all that's needed. Add nutrients and exercise, and you're on your way.

With every recipe, use salt and pepper to taste. Always use cold-pressed organic virgin oils. For cooking, use macadamia, coconut, and mustard. For all sauces, heat at a temperature that will not burn the food. Substitute rice or non-GMO soy milk for dairy like cheese, yogurt, and ice cream. Use gluten grains and flour for wheat. Feel free to be creative. You can exchange ingredients and add or subtract for taste as you like. To avoid chemicals from manufactured cookware, only use pots and pans made from stainless steel, glass, and iron. Never use aluminum.

Kalamata Olive Ratatouille

1 large onion, coarsely diced
2 cloves garlic, chopped
1 green pepper, chopped
1 medium eggplant, coarsely diced
1 zucchini, coarsely diced
1/2 cup Kalamata olives, pitted and halved
1 tablespoon safflower oil
2 tomatoes, coarsely diced, juice saved
1/2 teaspoon rosemary, chopped
1/2 teaspoon thyme, chopped
1 teaspoon basil, chopped
salt and pepper to taste

1. Saute the onion, zucchini, pepper, and eggplant in safflower oil on low heat until vegetables are soft.
2. Add the tomatoes and Kalamata olives and simmer for 10 minutes.
3. Add the rosemary, thyme, garlic, and basil.
4. Season with salt and pepper, and serve.

Chef's Notes:

This may be served on its own or with fish, tofu, or tempeh.

Mushroom Ragout with Walnuts and Prunes

Serves 4

1 cup shitake mushrooms, halved with stem removed and washed
1 cup crimi mushrooms, sliced with stem removed and washed
1 cup white mushrooms, sliced with stem removed and washed
1 cup maitake mushrooms, sliced with stem removed and washed
1 cup oyster mushrooms, halved with stem removed and washed
2 tablespoons safflower oil
1/2 cup prunes, pitted and split
1/2 cup walnuts, toasted
1 tablespoon tarragon, chopped
2 tablespoons walnut oil
1 medium onion, medium diced

1. Saute mushrooms and onions in oil until any moisture has evaporated. This should take about 10 minutes.
2. Add walnuts, prunes, tarragon, garlic, and walnut oil.
3. Season with pepper and serve hot or cold.

Chef's Notes:

You may use any combination of the above mushrooms or any other mushrooms. The objective is to include as many different mushrooms as possible.

Tempeh with Fennel, Turmeric, and Cumin Coulis

Serves 4

4 6-ounce tempeh filets
2 lemons, juiced
1/4 cup organic white wine

For the Coulis:
2 cups vegetable stock
1 teaspoon turmeric
1/2 teaspoon cumin seeds
2 heads fennel bulb, quartered, cored, and coarsely diced
1 teaspoon tarragon, chopped

1. Put stock, fennel, cumin, and turmeric in saucepan and simmer until fennel is tender.
2. Place this mixture in blender and blend until smooth.
3. Bake tempeh with lemon juice and wine on 350°F for 5 minutes.
4. Serve coulis with tempeh.

Chef's Notes:

"Coulis" is a term applied to pureed sauces.

Roasted Fall Root Vegetables

Serves 4

1 medium carrot, not peeled, washed and quartered
1 medium parsnip, washed and quartered and core removed
12 pearl onions, peeled
12 small heirloom potatoes (Russian fingerling, German butterball, ozette, yukon, or purple or red potatoes)
4 shallots, peeled
4 cloves garlic, peeled
1 small celery root peeled, coarsely diced
1/4 cup balsamic vinegar
1/4 cup maple syrup
1 teaspoon thyme
1/4 teaspoon coarse black pepper

1. Bake vegetables in a pan at 300°F for 30 to 45 minutes, making sure the potatoes are cooked.
2. Place in a bowl and toss with maple syrup, balsamic vinegar, thyme, and black pepper.
3. Return to pan and bake for 10 more minutes.
4. Remove and serve.

Marinated Cauliflower and Onions in Curry

1 head cauliflower, core removed and cut into florets
1 medium onion, peeled and ½-inch sliced
2 cloves garlic, peeled whole
2 teaspoons Madras Curry Powder
1/4 cup apple cider vinegar
1/4 cup rice syrup
1/2 cup water
2 whole bay leaves

1. Bring mixture of vinegar, rice syrup, water, and bay leaves to a simmer.
2. Add curry, garlic, onion, and cauliflower, simmer with lid on for 2 minutes.
3. Remove from heat, let cool in liquid at room temperature.
4. After 1 hour, place in refrigerator and serve chilled.

Chef's Notes:

You may substitute carrots for cauliflower or your favorite vegetable. I happen to enjoy how the flavor of curry combines with cauliflower.

Steamed Purple Potatoes with Basil

Serves 4

2 pounds purple potatoes, washed
2 cups whole basil leaves
1/3 cup extra virgin olive oil
coarse black pepper

1. Boil or steam potatoes until cooked but firm. Cut potatoes in half.
2. Place oil and basil in a blender and puree. Be careful not to over-blend.
3. Toss potatoes with basil oil and sprinkle with black pepper.

Chef's Notes:

This is a very simple but flavorful recipe. Use the freshest basil possible since it is the highlight of the dish.

Green Tea and Tamari with Bok Choy

    3 bags of green tea
    2 cups water
    1 tablespoon lemon grass, chopped
    1 clove garlic, crushed
    1/4 cup San-J Lite Tamari (soy)
    1 head bok choy, sliced and washed
    1 tablespoon toasted sesame oil

1. Bring water to boil and add tea, lemon grass, and garlic.
2. Steep the green tea bags for 5 minutes, then remove.
3. Return mixture to a boil and add the tamari and bok choy.
4. Cook bok choy until it just starts to soften.
5. Drizzle sesame oil on the bok choy and serve hot.

Chef's Notes:

Feel free to add other vegetables such as onions or broccoli. Serving suggestion: serve hot with tamari-tea.

Apple Jicama and Cumin Salad

Serves 4

2 Granny Smith apples, cored, medium diced with skin
1 medium jicama, skinned, medium diced
1 teaspoon ground cumin
3 scallions, chopped lightly
1 red bell pepper, medium diced
1 tablespoon mint, chopped lightly
1/3 cup Basic Vinaigrette (see page 159)
1/4 teaspoon turmeric

Mix all ingredients and serve.

Chef's Notes:

Use a small electric coffee grinder to grind spices. Cumin, fennel seed, coriander, allspice, cinnamon, and any other spices work well.

Celeriac and Orange Salad

Serves 4

2 cups celeriac root, peeled and medium diced
3 scallions, chopped
2 oranges, juiced
1/4 teaspoon ground cardamom
1/4 teaspoon coarse ground black pepper
1 tablespoon mint, lightly chopped
2 oranges, peeled and sliced
1/3 cup Basic Vinaigrette (see recipe on opposite page)

Mix all ingredients in a bowl and serve.

Basic Vinaigrette

    1/2 cup apple cider vinegar
    4 tablespoons dijon mustard
    1 tablespoons tahini
    4 tablespoons honey
    2 cloves garlic, peeled
    1 cup expeller-pressed sunflower oil
    1/4 cup extra virgin olive oil
    1/2 cup walnut oil
    2 tablespoons flax oil
    1 tablespoon parsley, lightly chopped
    1 tablespoon thyme, lightly chopped
    1 tablespoon rosemary, lightly chopped
    ground white pepper to taste

1. Blend vinegar, mustard, tahini, honey, and garlic in a blender.
2. While blending slowly drizzle all the oils in. This will cause the vinaigrette to become creamy.
3. After all the oil has been incorporated add the thyme, rosemary, and parsley. Season with white pepper to taste.

Super Healthy Vinaigrette

Make the Basic Vinaigrette (see recipe on page 159), but add the following ingredients at the end:
10–20 drops pau d'arco tincture, alcohol-free
10–20 drops milk thistle tincture, alcohol-free
10–20 drops burdock tincture, alcohol-free
2–4 drops essential oil of rosemary
2–4 drops essential oil of thyme
2–4 drops essential oil of basil

Add one or all of these ingredients for added benefits.

Mushroom Salad with Burdock Vinaigrette

2 tablespoons coconut oil
1 cup shiitake mushrooms, stemmed, quartered, and washed
1 cup white mushrooms, stemmed, sliced, and washed
1 cup portabello mushrooms, stemmed, gills removed, sliced, and washed
1 large onion, medium diced
1 clove garlic, chopped
1 stalk burdock, whole
1/2 cup Basic Vinaigrette (on page 159), plus 20 drops burdock tincture

1. Cook all mushrooms in sauté pan with oil on low. Cook until mushrooms are soft and any excess water has evaporated and let cool.
2. Wash and scrub burdock, then grate or thinly slice.
3. Add to mushrooms to the vinaigrette with burdock slices. Serve warm or cold. It is best to let marinate for 4 to 36 hours.

Curried Lentils

Serves 4

1 cup French lentils, sorted and rinsed
2 teaspoons curry powder
1 teaspoon safflower oil
6 cups water
1 medium onion, finely diced
1/4 cup raisins
2 apples, finely diced
1 tablespoons apple cider vinegar
3 tablespoons untoasted sesame oil
1 teaspoon basil, lightly chopped

1. Bring 6 cups of water to a boil, then add lentils and boil for 25 minutes until lentils are firm but cooked. Then drain and rinse them under clean water.
2. Toast curry powder in a pan in the oven at 350°F for 5 minutes.
3. Add toasted sesame oil in a sauté pan and gently cook onions until soft. After the onions are cooked, add them to the lentils along with curry, raisins, apples, vinegar, coconut oil, and basil.

Kombu Noodles with Sesame

Serves 4

8 ounces kombu noodles, cooked
1/2 cup green bell pepper, medium diced
1/4 cup red onion, medium diced
3 scallions, sliced
1 teaspoon ginger, chopped
1 teaspoon sesame seeds
2 tablespoons Braggs Liquid Aminos
2 tablespoons toasted sesame oil

Mix all ingredients and serve.

Chef's Notes:

Kombu noodles can be purchased in health or in Asian food stores' frozen section.

Corn, Fennel, and Mushrooms

Serves 4

1 cup frozen corn kernels thawed, cooked, and cooled
2 fennel bulbs, thinly sliced, core removed
8 ounces white mushrooms, stemmed, washed, cooked, and cooled
8 ounces shiitake mushrooms, stemmed, washed, cooked, and cooled
1/2 cup Basic or Super Healthy Vinaigrette (recipes on page 159, 160)
1 tablespoons tarragon, chopped lightly
1 teaspoon thyme, chopped
1 teaspoon parsley, chopped lightly

Mix all ingredients together and serve.

Soybeans with Green Onions and Sesame

Serves 4

4 cups soybeans, fresh or frozen, cooked and cooled
6 scallions, sliced
2 tablespoons sesame oil
1 teaspoon mint, lightly chopped
1 tablespoon Braggs Liquid Aminos
4 teaspoons lemon juice
2 tablespoons sesame seeds
1 clove garlic
1 teaspoon dulse flakes

Combine all ingredients and serve.

Potato and Nettle Salad

Serves 4

1 pound yukon potatoes, 1-inch cubed
3 scallions, sliced
2 cups nettle leaves, washed
1/2 cup Basic Vinaigrette (on page 159)

1. Place potatoes in a pot of cold water and bring them to a simmer. Cook potatoes for about 15 to 20 minutes. Prick potatoes with a paring knife to check for doneness.
2. Cool the potatoes in cool water and drain.
3. Bring 1 pint of water to boil and cook nettles for 5 seconds.
4. Strain nettles and shock in an ice water bath. Next, chop the nettles lightly.
5. Mix all ingredients in a bowl and serve.

Heirloom Tomatoes

Serves 4

4 to 8 heirloom tomatoes, sliced
1 tablespoon basil, lightly chopped
1/4 cup extra virgin olive oil

Slice tomatoes and line them up on an oversized plate, top with basil and olive oil.

Chef's Notes:

The dish works best when tomatoes are in season in your geographic area. Select tomatoes that are ripe and full of flavor. Most tomatoes will work, but any heirloom variety is preferred. Do not be discouraged by the appearance of heirloom tomatoes, they are usually full of flavor.

Also, never refrigerate a tomato. Room temperature tomatoes taste and store better.

Three Bean and Oregano Salad

1/2 cup kidney beans, cooked
1 cup white beans, cooked
1/2 cup Anasazi beans, cooked
1/2 cup Basic Vinaigrette (on page 159)
2 tablespoons oregano, lightly chopped
1 clove garlic, peeled and chopped

Mix all ingredients. This dish can be saved for up to three days.

Chef's Notes:

Any beans will work, even the addition of a fresh green bean.

Purslane and White Beans

Serves 4

2 cups white beans, cooked
1 cup purslane leaves, chopped
1 teaspoon rosemary, chopped
2 cloves garlic, chopped
4 tablespoons basil, lightly chopped
1 tablespoon Italian parsley, lightly chopped
1/4 teaspoon coarsely ground black pepper
1 tablespoon balsamic vinegar
1 tablespoon apple cider vinegar
1/4 cup walnut oil
1/4 cup extra virgin olive oil

Mix all ingredients and serve chilled.

Bean Cassoulet with Herb Sprout Crumbs

Serves 4

1 tablespoon macadamia nut oil
2 medium onions, finely diced
2 cloves garlic, chopped
1 green bell pepper, finely diced
1 cup white beans, cooked
1 cup kidney beans, cooked
1 cup garbanzo beans, cooked
1 large tomato, diced
1 teaspoon thyme, chopped
1 teaspoon basil, lightly chopped
1 teaspoon rosemary, chopped
1 teaspoon parsley, lightly chopped
3 slices fresh multigrain bread
3 tablespoons extra virgin olive oil

1. Heat macadamia nut oil in oil on low in sauté pan and cook onions, peppers, and garlic until soft. Add beans, tomato, 3/4 teaspoon thyme, 3/4 teaspoon basil, and 3/4 teaspoon rosemary. Heat thoroughly.
2. Place bean mixture in casserole dish.
3. Take bread and puree in food processor with rest of herbs and 1 tablespoon of olive oil.
4. Top beans with bread crumbs and bake at 375°F for 20 minutes until bread crumbs are toasted.
5. Remove and drizzle with remaining olive oil.

Potato Nettle Soup

Serves 4

1 pound yukon potatoes, washed and coarsely diced
3 cups vegetable stock
1/2 medium onion, chopped
2 cups nettle leaves, washed
salt and pepper to taste

1. Slow simmer potatoes and onions in vegetable stock until cooked.
2. Add nettle leaves and cook for 1 minute.
3. Place in blender and puree until smooth.

Miso with Lettuce Soup

Serves 4

1 medium onion, finely diced
4 cloves garlic, chopped
1 pound firm tofu, medium diced
6 cups vegetable stock
2 teaspoons ginger, chopped
3 scallions, sliced
1 tablespoon cilantro, lightly chopped
3 tablespoons basil, lightly chopped
1 tablespoons mint, lightly chopped
3 tablespoons white miso
3 cups greens (romaine, spinach, chard), sliced very thinly
To taste: mixed seaweed, hijiki, kombu, kelp, and nori

1. Simmer onion, garlic, tofu, ginger, and seaweed in vegetable stock for 5 minutes.
2. Add miso, scallions, cilantro, basil, mint, and greens, and serve.

Chef's Notes:

You should never simmer miso, so always add miso to the recipe after the cooking process is done. There are several types of miso available, experiment and use the one you like best.

Potato, Corn, and Cashew Soup

Serves 4

1 pound yukon potatoes, washed and halved
5 cups vegetable stock
1/2 cups cashews
1 medium onion, diced
1 clove garlic, peeled
1 cup rice milk
1/2 teaspoon thyme, chopped
1/2 cup corn kernels, cooked

1. Cook potatoes, onions, cashews, and garlic in stock until tender. This should take around 30 minutes. Add soymilk and thyme.
2. In a blender, puree mixture until smooth.
3. Add corn and return to simmer for 1 minute.

Chef's Notes:

Always choose the smallest possible potatoes available. Pound for pound, smaller potatoes have much more skin. The skin has a lot of flavor and more concentrated nutrients.

Mushroom and Miso Soup

1 medium onion, medium diced
4 cloves garlic, chopped
2 cups mixed mushrooms (shiitake, miatake, oyster, woodear, white, or brown), washed and cut into bite-size pieces
6 cups vegetable stock
1 tablespoon light miso
2 teaspoons Braggs Liquid Aminos
1 tablespoon dulse flakes
3 tablespoons basil, lightly chopped
2 teaspoons cilantro, lightly chopped
4 scallions, sliced

1. Gently simmer onions, garlic, and mushrooms in vegetable stock for 8 to 10 minutes.
2. Add miso, Braggs, dulse flakes, basil, cilantro, and scallions.
3. Serve.

Chef's Notes:

Tofu would make a simple addition.

Puree of Carrot and Fennel Soup

Serves 4

1 bulb fennel, chopped with core removed
2 large carrots, washed and chopped
5 cups vegetable stock
1 bay leaf
1 sprig thyme
1 teaspoon fennel seeds
1 cup soy milk or rice milk
1 cup honey

1. Simmer fennel, carrots, bay leaf, fennel seeds, and thyme in vegetable stock until vegetables are tender.
2. Add honey and the soy or rice milk. Then, in a blender, puree all ingredients until smooth.

Cold Potato Spinach and Nettle Soup

    1 pound yukon potatoes, washed and halved
    1 medium onion, diced
    4 cups vegetable stock
    1 clove garlic, peeled
    2 cups spinach, washed and loosely packed
    2 cups nettle leaves, washed and loosely packed
    2 cups soy milk or rice milk

1. Cook potatoes, onions, and garlic in stock until tender. This should take around 30 minutes.
2. Add spinach and nettles and simmer for two more minutes. Add soy milk and thyme.
3. In a blender, puree all ingredients until smooth.
4. Let soup cool and serve.

Chef's Notes:

Always choose the smallest potatoes possible. Also, leftover cooked salmon would make a great addition to this soup.

Vegan French Onion Soup

Serves 4

6 cups vegetarian stock
2 large onions, peeled, split, and 1/4-inch sliced
2 cloves garlic, chopped
4 slices fresh multigrain bread, toasted and cut into quarters
4 slices vegetarian Swiss cheese
1 teaspoon thyme, chopped
2 teaspoons Braggs Liquid Aminos

1. Divide sliced onions into thirds, take 1/3 of onions and roast them in an oven at 425°F for 20 to 30 minutes. The onions should turn brown without burning.
2. Bring the stock to a boil and add the roasted onions and 1/3 more raw onions. Simmer for 10 minutes.
3. Add the last 1/3 of onions and turn off the heat.
4. Add thyme and Braggs Liquid Aminos.
5. Ladle soup into ovenproof crocks, add bread, and then cover the bread with the Swiss cheese.
6. Place into broiler until cheese melts and browns. Serve immediately.

Buckwheat Soba with Pecans and Vegetables

Serves 2–3

1 7-ounce package soba noodles, cooked according to label
1 cup pecan halves or pieces
2 cloves garlic, chopped
1/2 cup onions, 1-inch diced
1/2 cup celery, 1-inch diced
1/2 cup carrots, 1-inch diced
1 cup broccoli florets
1/2 cup shiitake mushrooms, stem removed, washed, and sliced
1/2 cup Chinese cabbage, shredded
1/2 cup bell peppers, 1-inch diced

For the Sauce:
3 tablespoons peanut butter, natural
1 tablespoons toasted sesame oil
1 tablespoon Braggs Liquid Aminos
1/2 cup vegetable stock
1 tablespoon cilantro

1. In a blender, blend in all the ingredients for sauce.
2. Steam onions, celery, carrots, broccoli, shiitakes, cabbage, and peppers until just cooked.
3. Bring sauce to a simmer and add pecans, soba, garlic, and vegetables.

Broccoli Rabe with Brown Rice Penne, Garlic, and Extra Virgin Oil

Serves 4

1/2 pound brown rice penne, cooked
1/2 cup vegetable stock
1 bunch broccoli rabe, washed
1 tablespoon toasted sesame oil
4 cloves garlic, chopped
3 tablespoons extra virgin olive oil
1 tablespoons parsley, lightly chopped
1 tablespoons basil, lightly chopped

1. Cook broccoli rabe by boiling in water for 1 to 3 minutes.
2. In a sauté pan, add oil and cook garlic on low for 1 to 3 minutes.
3. Add penne, broccoli rabe, and vegetable stock.
4. Serve and drizzle olive oil, parsley, and basil.

Tempeh and Kidney Bean Chili

1 tablespoon hot sesame oil
1/2 medium onion, finely diced
1/2 jalapeno chile, finely diced
4 cloves garlic, chopped
1/2 teaspoon cumin
4 tablespoons chili seasoning (no salt and nonirradiated)
4 tablespoons tomato puree
1 cup dry kidney beans, soaked overnight in 3 cups of water
1 2- to 3-inch piece kelp
4 cups vegetable stock (reserve 1 cup for chili)
4 tablespoons black strap molasses

1. Rinse beans and bring them to a simmer with stock and kelp. Cook beans until they are tender but still keep their shape.
2. In a soup pot on low heat add the oil.
3. Gently cook onion, garlic, and jalapeno until tender.
4. Add tempeh, cumin, tomato puree, molasses, chili seasoning, and beans.
5. Add vegetable stock if necessary.
6. Cook slowly for 20 minutes and serve.

Pasta e Fagioli

Serves 2–4

1/2 pound quinoa pasta, cooked
1/2 cup white beans, soaked
3 cups vegetable stock
1 2- to 3-inch piece kelp
1/2 cup celery, medium diced
1/2 cup carrots, medium diced
1 cup onions, medium diced
1 sprig rosemary
1 sprig thyme
1 bay leaf
4 cloves garlic, crushed

1. Rinse beans after soaking, bring beans and vegetable stock to a simmer. Remove any foam that forms on top during the cooking process.
2. Add kelp, thyme, rosemary, bay leaf, garlic, onions, celery, and carrots. Cook beans until tender while they are still holding their shape.
3. When beans are cooked, add cooked pasta.
4. If beans have absorbed all the stock, simply add more until the desired consistency.

Apple, Walnut, and Tofu Salad

Serves 2

1/4 cup onions, minced
1/4 cup celery, minced
2 teaspoons raw apple cider vinegar
1/2 cup Nayonaise
1/4 teaspoons ground cumin
1 apple, medium diced
1 pound firm tofu, drained and crumbled
1/4 cup raw walnuts

1. Combine onions, celery, vinegar, Nayonaise, cumin, and apple and mix well.
2. Mix in tofu and walnuts. Serve or refrigerate for up to 3 days.

Fennel and Pecan Salad

Serves 2

1 cup fennel root, sliced
1/2 cups dandelion greens, well packed
1/2 cup Italian parsley leaves, well packed
1/2 cup fresh peaches, well packed
1/4 cup pecans, well packed
1 cup pomegranate seeds (optional)

1. Combine the fennel, dandelion greens, parsley, and peaches in a large salad bowl.
2. Toss with a light, sweet salad dressing or vinaigrette of your choice and top with the pecan and pomegranate seeds. Serve chilled.

Pretty Parfait

Serves 4 to 6

1 cup fresh pineapple (if canned, use unsweetened and drain)
1 cup papaya
1/2 cup raspberries, fresh or frozen (without sugar)
raisins and walnuts for garnish
nondairy whipped cream

1. Place the pineapple in the blender and puree. Pour into a bowl. Puree the papaya the same way.
2. Using a parfait glass or any clear dessert glass or cup, pour in pineapple till the glass is one-quarter full. Now pour or spoon in papaya puree till the glass is half full. Continue layering.
3. Top with fresh raspberries and the raisins and walnuts. Serve as is or chill and serve—chilling improves the flavor. Swirl whipped cream on top.

Curry Chickpeas

Serves 2

12 ounces (1 can) chickpeas
1 cup water
3 tablespoons toasted sesame oil
1/2 cup onion, finely chopped
4 cloves garlic
2 scallions, sliced
1 teaspoon ginger, freshly grated
3 tablespoons lemon juice
1/4 cup roasted pecans
4 tablespoons ground curry
sea salt to taste
radicchio, finely chopped, for garnish (optional)
fresh green salad (pre-mixed available in grocery stores)

1. Simmer chickpeas in water with sesame oil, onions, garlic, scallions, ginger, and lemon juice for 15 to 20 minutes, until chickpeas are soft.
2. Add pecans, cumin, and salt. Let cook 5 or more minutes. Be careful not to overcook, or it will become mushy. Drain.
3. Garnish with radicchio or cilantro and serve with a fresh green salad. Serve immediately.

Eggplant Mozzarella

Serves 2

2 medium eggplants, peeled
sea salt to taste
4 tablespoons EVOO blended with 2 sprigs chopped saffron
2/3 cup tofu cream cheese
1/4 pound fresh soy mozzarella, thinly sliced
8 ounces (1 can) tomato sauce
1 teaspoon dried tarragon
1/4 teaspoon cayenne pepper
2 tablespoons fresh basil, chopped
1/4 cup rice or soy Parmesan cheese

1. Cut eggplant into slices ¼ inch thick. Sprinkle slices with salt and weight them down with a heavy plate.
2. Let stand for 1 hour or overnight. Drain and rinse slices and pat them dry.
3. Mix chopped basil into tofu cream cheese.
4. In a heavy skillet, heat oil over medium heat. Sauté eggplant slices until golden brown on both sides. Drain on paper towel.
5. Preheat oven to 350°F.
6. In a round casserole dish, layer eggplant, tofu cream cheese mixture, soy mozzarella, tomato sauce, oregano, and cayenne. Continue to build layers until you have used up all of the ingredients. The final layer should be tofu cream cheese mixture sprinkled with Parmesan.
7. Bake for 20 minutes, until top is golden brown and bubbly. Serve warm.

You Gotta Love It

Serves 3 to 4

1 cup finely chopped chard, steamed 5 minutes
1 cup pears, diced
1 cup mushrooms, sliced
1/2 cup leeks, sliced
1 teaspoon sea salt
1 teaspoon freshly ground black pepper
2 tablespoons EVOO
4 1/2 teaspoons apple juice
1/2 cup black-eyed peas, steamed 15 minutes
1/2 teaspoon paprika (preferably Hungarian)
3 tablespoons ground allspice
1 teaspoon ground nutmeg
1/2 cup cashews

1. In a large saucepan, sauté chard, pears, mushrooms, leeks, salt, and pepper in oil over medium-high heat for 7 minutes.
2. Add remaining ingredients and cook an additional 10 minutes.
3. Serve hot.

Indian Casserole

Serves 2

2 1/2 tablespoons coconut oil, divided
1/4 cup oat flour
1/2 cup cooked split peas
1/3 cup curry powder
1/4 teaspoon minced garlic
1/4 teaspoon sea salt
1/4 teaspoon oregano
1/4 cup filtered water
1/2 cup kale, coarsely chopped
1/2 cup broccoli, chopped into bite-size pieces
1 cup brown short-grain rice, cooked
1/2 avocado, sliced

1. Preheat oven to 375°F. Lightly grease 4-by-8-inch baking pan with coconut oil.
2. In a blender, combine oat flour, split peas, oil, curry, garlic, sea salt, oregano, and water.
3. In a separate bowl, combine kale, broccoli, and brown rice. Mix well.
4. Transfer to covered baking pan, top with flour and peas mixture. Bake for 15 minutes. Place avocado slices on top for garnish.
5. Serve hot.

Vegetable Stir Fry

Serves 4

2 tomatoes (to render 1/2 cup juice)
1 cut extra-firm tofu, cut into 1-inch cubes
2 tablespoons olive oil
1 cup yellow onions, chopped
2 cups frozen peas
1 cup tomatoes, chopped
3/4 cup plain soy milk
3 teaspoons apple cider vinegar
1/2 cup arugula, finely chopped
2 green chili peppers, finely chopped
3 cloves garlic, crushed
2 teaspoons ginger root, grated
1 teaspoon ground coriander
1 teaspoon ground turmeric
1/4 teaspoon chili powder
1 1/2 teaspoons sea salt
spinach or other leafy green salad

1. Juice tomatoes. Set aside 1/2 cup of the juice.
2. In a large frying pan, brown tofu in oil over high heat.
3. Add onions. Sauté 2 to 3 minutes, or until onions are soft.
4. Reduce heat to medium-low. Add the 1/2 cup of tomato juice and remaining ingredients except the salad, and simmer uncovered for 5 minutes.
5. Serve with fresh green salad.

• CHAPTER 9 •

Love

In 1943 psychologist Abraham Maslow created his Hierarchy of Needs, a pyramid-shaped diagram separating all human needs into layers that each person needs to build in order to become a self-actualized person. In other words, Maslow provided a checklist of the building blocks for a full life.

There are five layers in the pyramid, and it is necessary for an individual to secure the bottom four levels of needs before they can become a fully actualized person. An actualized person is ideally devoid of anxiety since all needs have been met, and he or she will have the ability to be a moral, creative, resourceful, and responsible human being.

At the bottom level are our base physiological human needs: breathing, food, water, sleep, homeostasis, and excretion. These are merely the foundational needs to live; without them we cannot. The next level up are safety requirements, such as security of the body, shelter, employment, keeping healthy, and being able to provide for your family. These needs are those that secure livelihood, irrespective of the quality of that livelihood. We all know that you can have a good job and food on the table, but your mood will still end up in the dumps from time to time. That's where the next two layers come in.

Love and esteem are our higher needs in life and what we need to feel fully complete. Their layers in Maslow's pyramid intertwine; it's very difficult to have one without the other. Our love needs encompass friendships, family relationships, and sexual intimacy, while our esteem needs are having the self-esteem and confidence to gain respect from others and ourselves. On the road towards becoming a fully realized being we need friendships and family connections, which can help us build the self-confidence and esteem necessary to begin and keep a healthy romantic relationship.

Think about your last unsuccessful relationship (unless you're fortunate enough not to have one). Were you happy during most of the relationship, gaining benefits from your partner, or was the relationship filled with you or your partner's egotistical needs, where you would push on each other to act a certain way or do certain things? Were you supporting and complementing each other rather than seeking to fulfill your mutual selfish needs?

Often, when an individual enters a relationship before becoming more self-actualized, he will seek out his missing needs through his partner. And this can happen in a multitude of ways. If a man is not confident, he may sarcastically insult his girlfriend, hoping to bring her down to his level. Or he may require her to stroke his ego with compliments while failing to return the favor. When people are depressed or anxious, they may fail to see and meet their partner's needs since they are too wrapped up in their own problems. Then when the relationship ends, they are surprised and become further depressed by feeling alone. We must learn to think of relationships as beautiful opportunities from which to grow, not as support systems, which can drag each other down.

Love can be a wonderful experience—a powerful state of being that we seek all of our lives. When we have love, it picks up our day. The lack of love can be a burden, a feeling of emptiness in our lives. Yet it is important to be a confident individual who is capable of loving *before* entering in a relationship. And once you're in a loving, caring relationship, you've got one of the best weapons against anxiety and depression you can have.

Now I know building the confidence to begin a relationship can be hard, especially if you're recovering from anxiety and depression. Using the protocols, diet change, positive thinking, and exercise outlined in the previous chapters can help you move up the pyramid of self-actualization. There will always be setbacks if you perceive them as setbacks. In today's image-conscious society, it's easy to see attractive people on television and give up your diet and exercise since your health goals feel so far away. But stick with it. Lifestyle changes are difficult, but their rewards are worth it.

If you've found yourself in an unhappy relationship, sit down and think about whether or not it's healthy for you. A good relationship can help life's day-to-day trials go by easier, but an unhealthy relationship can slowly drain your energy and happiness. If you are with an abusive partner, assess for yourself whether it's worth it to stick through your lover's abuse. There's no shame in walking away from an unhealthy relationship. Sometimes it's better to go on your own and free yourself to find the love you desire with another mate.

If you decide that this damaged relationship is worth saving, there are several things you can try to salvage it. Have an open discourse with your partner discussing your problems. Listen to each other patiently and really try to hear your partner's needs. This can be hard to do without getting into arguments and at first many men are hesitant to be open about their feelings. Couple's therapy can be the route you choose, since having a patient, healing conversation could be easier for some people when they have a moderator.

For some people it's hard to open up face-to-face with their partners. Now that's something that needs to change over time for a healthy relationship to evolve, but there's something that these people can do to begin open dialogues with their partners.

Love

A study at the University of Texas tested the effects of expressive writing between partners. They took a group of 86 couples and for three consecutive days asked them to perform the simple task of writing down either their deepest thoughts or feelings about their relationship or their daily activities. The couples who wrote down their thoughts were much more likely to be together three and six months in the future.

Furthermore, a review of the couples' text messages also showed more predictors of a healthy, long relationship. Partners who texted more frequently stayed together longer. In the healthiest relationships partners would joke around with each other and give excited details of their daily lives, while unhealthy couples merely sent updates for when they were running late or no messages at all. Couples with more interactivity stayed stronger longer.

So what you and your partner can do is sit down and write out notes of your own deepest thoughts and feelings. You don't have to do this together, or even at the same time, but doing this several times for one week can help you start a discourse between each other. You may learn things about your partner you never knew, like about their beliefs of your relationship and feelings he or she has. You might even learn something about your own feelings in the process. Hopefully over time you two can feel more comfortable with each other and have a happy, supportive rapport—one where you two keep each other strong against the stresses in the world instead of hiding from the stresses of each other.

And a good, communicative relationship will be a huge asset in your fight against depression. Throughout many studies, partners in healthy relationships show lower levels of anxiety across the board. They are also more likely not to smoke or drink as much, finding solace in each other rather than through vices. Couples together for longer periods of time often show healthier cardiovascular symptoms. This is also helped by the fact that wine and dark chocolate, often used as gifts for lovers, help promote a healthier heart when consumed in moderation.

Another benefit of relationships is that hugs, cuddling, and kisses help to ward off anxiety. In the last few years scientists have been looking into a hormone called oxytocin and its stress-relieving properties. Oxytocin runs throughout your body, but mostly resides in your brain. It gets pumped out when you receive physical pleasure, like a physiological reward system for receiving positive touch. This powerful hormone accomplishes a lot in your body by improving your mood and lowering the level of stress hormones. It also reduces blood pressure, raises our tolerance for pain, and helps you heal faster. So being in a healthy relationship with healthy levels of affection can actually make you a stronger person.

Love is one of the strongest forces in our world and can be both a source and relief from anxiety and depression. By learning to be a full person you can reap the benefits of a caring, mutually supportive relationship, but if you enter a commitment seeking needs out from your partner the relationship can eat away at both of your lives. Remember, you live for yourself, not for the other person. You are with them because you want them in your life, not because you need them to be happy. And once you've found love, what else can you ask for?

• CHAPTER 10 •

Experts Speak Out

Here's a collection of quotes from leading experts in the fields of biology, psychology, and spirituality, where they share what they've learned over years of helping others.

Dr. Lester Sauvage, M.D., Professor Emeritus of Surgery University of Washington

A little stress tunes us out, but too much can be deadly.

Barbara Biziou, Author of The Joy of Family Friends

Stress to me is anything that takes you away from a calm center. And it's not necessarily what happens in your life, it's your attitude towards what happens in your life.

Bruce Lipton, Ph.D., Cellular Biologist

My research, which started about 1967, I was studying stem cells. What I did, I put stem cells in a culture dish. What I would do, I would create a culture dish of genetically identical cells, change the culture medium, which is the environment for the cells, and with the culture medium I changed the cells or fate of the cells, their genetic activity. This influence of the environment on changing genes is called epigenetics. Well, I'm doing this in a Petri dish with stem cells. We must understand a very important fact. That a human being is the equivalent of a skin covered Petri dish. A human has about fifty trillion cells growing within their body and the growing media inside the body is called the blood. By changing the chemical composition of the blood, I am influencing the genetic composition of the cells. Whether I do it in a plastic dish, or I do it in a skin-covered body, it's still the influence of the environment affecting the genetic readout. Here's where the issue connects in regard to love and fear and our lives. The blood is the culture medium of the body's cells, and if I change the composition of the blood, then I change the fate of the cells. Well the question is what changes the composition of the blood? The answer is the brain. The brain changes the composition of the blood. And the brain controls that chemistry of the blood in regard to our chemistry of life. So if I feel love, I release a different chemistry in my brain than if I'm in fear. For example, if I'm in love I release oxytocin, serotonin, and growth hormones. These chemicals in the blood cause the growth and enhancement of the health of cells, whether it's in a human body, or in a plastic dish. In contrast, when I'm in fear, I release stress hormones like cortisol and norepinephrine, or a histamine. Those chemicals actually change the fate of the cells and put the cells in a protection posture. So it comes down to very simply this. Our attitudes, or our perceptions of the environment, whether it includes love, or whether it includes fear, it changes the blood, via the action of the brain, and the chemistry of the blood changes the genetics of our cells, epigenetics. So therefore it's very important what you perceive in life because your perceptions are actually altering and directly influencing your gene activity, and there is a very profound difference in the chemistry of a person who is in love, and the chemistry of a person who has fear, so it really is incumbent on us to recognize that our emotions, and attitudes, and responses to our environment are controlling our genetics via the chemistry of the blood.

During our programming as children, we really observe from our parents and the community around us what we should be doing to become an active and contributing part of our society. And unfortunately our teachers have not been very good in that regard, because it's really been a whole series of lessons on self-gratification and self-serving and me versus you and unfortunately this is the wrong tact, this is not what evolution is all about. The way we have to correct his trap, is we have to get out of the old reactive behavior patterns and we have to start generating new behaviors until we really start to understand the nature of love and harmony, and feelings that we get, and the result of those feelings of being in love and harmony that we will ultimately start to let go of the old beliefs and focus on the new one. And it's very interesting because as a large percent of the population is trying to awaken at this point, awaken to a better understanding of life, a better understanding of health, we find that the media and the religious sources around us are trying to hold us back, and the reason why is because when we become awakened, we become empowered. And the last number of hundreds of years on this planet, the powers to be recognized that they are not being awakened, they control us. And as we start to awaken now, their fear of losing power over us keeps pushing the old story in front of us, the old images. The war, the competition, the battling, rather than give us the images of what is better than what we have, what is a future we can thrive into. It really is incumbent upon us as individuals to take that power back for ourselves, because once we do, not only do we create harmony and love in our life, but physiologically we become healthy, and grow, and have a wonderful experience of living in this garden called Earth.

During our development, we start to acquire patterns of behavior and programs that reflect the environment that we're in. So if I grew up in a family, where let's say there was an abusive parent, and everyday I started receiving this abuse, whether it's verbal or physical, I begin to develop a program expecting this kind of activity every day. It's like a habit. So every day I'm looking forward towards feeding this habit through an abusive parent, so why this becomes important as we get older and we still have a habit of looking for this in our life, if we meet up with other people, we would expect them to fulfill and live out the habit that we've acquired. So that, if I was abused by my parents when I was a child and now I'm getting older then I'm looking to maintain this abusive relationship in my life. Therefore, even if my partner isn't willing to be that abusive, I will actually seek it in order to create a fulfillment of a habit. It's an urge to actually end up experiencing what you're used to experiencing. So if you're used to that kind of unfortunate background you will actually try to create a future that will have the same emotional and physiological characteristics and seek abuse.

The biggest problem reprogramming the subconscious mind is that we've held some kind of belief that if we become consciously aware of something, then I have profoundly influenced the program of the subconscious mind, and this is where the problem arises because there is this disconnect that we suppose lies between the two minds. One is the equivalent of a tape recorder and the other is the conscious mind, the creative mind. I have a new idea in my creative, conscious life. I want to create love, I want to create harmony, I want to share my life with all these people in this community, and the question is just because I acquired this in my conscious mind, did I in any way influence the programming of the subconscious mind, and the answer in not really, and the reason is this. The subconscious mind is more like a machine, like a tape player. Here's a simple story, an analogy. I have a program in a tape player, I push play and the program repeats, and every time I push play it repeats the same program. Imagine if you didn't like the program. How much talking and yelling at the tape player will it take before the tape changes? And the answer is, it will never change that way. The significance is this. You can change the tape, but there are processes like pushing the record button that will engage the new tape information to be overwritten on the old program. My point: just because our conscious becomes aware of another way, a better way of life, it in no way impacts the original programming. We must do processing to get this programming in, so if you understand the processes and characteristics of how the subconscious mind learns and then use that learning process, then we are more able to effectively change the program, but the most important thing is this. Just because our conscious mind sees that the program isn't good and we talk to ourselves, did that talking change the program? And the answer is no. The biggest part of this problem is being aware of where you want to go and still find yourself repeating the same limiting, self-sabotaging program even though your conscious mind is aware of another way of life.

In today's world, we're really focused on the types of information we receive from our leaders and our teachers, and frequently we begin to realize this information isn't very supportive of the lives of others on this planet. So the question is, what it is we can do in the face of programming that is personally limiting and sabotaging or negative in the world that we're living. The most important thing we can understand is that we must start operating from a level of consciousness and let go of the automatic subconscious programming. With consciousness we are empowered to create the world that we want. The subconscious mind is basically just filled with programs primarily downloaded from other people, So when we're operating from our subconscious mind we're not necessarily fulfilling what we want in our lives, we're fulfilling the programs of other people. So if we want to change, then it's incumbent on us to know that we must start acting consciously. Be here now. Pay attention to what is going on, because in the moment of now, you have absolute control. Now, a very interesting point about this, is the relationship when people fall very deeply in love, and why I bring this up is, there's a period called the honeymoon. And the honeymoon period is, if you ask anyone who's deeply engaged in a very active honeymoon, are you healthy, and they say yes, do you have energy, and they say yes, I say how's your world, and they would say it's heaven on Earth, everything is beautiful, and everything is wonderful, and before that honeymoon period runs out, they realize this. When a person is fully in love they're actually creating heaven on Earth. When the honeymoon ends, it's because the subconscious programming of others begins to interfere with our lives, and the relationship starts to fall apart. My point about this is very simple. When we're on our honeymoon, it's because we are not relying on our subconscious programs, we're relying on our conscious creativity. So the question is do you want to create heaven on Earth? The answer is yes. Well then we have to acquire that ability to get back into conscious control, just like we were in when fell in love, because that's when we created heaven on Earth. And so it's important to recognize, a, we can do it, and have done so many times in our lives, and b, make it an active process on our part to not rely on the subconscious programming, but to actually take control of our lives using our conscious belief system.

When we have been misprogrammed and really can't respond properly to the concept of love and harmony and beauty in the world that we live in, we have to recognize that those programs are downloaded into our subconscious mind. Our subconscious mind is basically the equivalent of a tape recorder. It records a program and every time you press play you get the same program back. Well until we get out of that subconscious mind, we become a victim of those programs. Well the question is, how do we get out of this, and the problem is, how do we understand the power of the conscious mind. It's the conscious mind that can override the subconscious mind. Unfortunately the conscious mind which is the creative mind, the mind that has our wishes, our desires, your aspirations, this mind on a general day-to-day basis operates only 5 percent of the time. So basically it says that 95 percent of our day we are unconsciously operating from programs that have been prerecorded into our subconscious mind, but for personal empowerment, we need to be able to emphasize our conscious mind, because that's the one that can come out of subconscious programming. The biggest effort of ours in this world is to correct the misprogramming of our youth and put into our lives much more healthy, harmonizing, loving programs that we can reprogram in the subconscious mind, using the conscious mind.

Paul McGhee, Ph.D., Author of Health, Healing, and the Amuse System

The pace of change in our lives, especially in the workplace, it just continues to increase. And so people are asked to do more with less. You have to do things faster. There's the information explosion. People cannot keep up with the amount of things they have to learn to keep their job because it keeps changing, and so the bar keeps being raised high. That's a phrase heard in the workplace often. Whatever work you did last year, next year you have to do more.

Neill Raff, M.D., Complementary Internal Medicine

There's a great expression called floating anxiety. People who have chronic anxiety have this little black cloud floating over their heads, like unemployed anxiety.

Dr. Michael Wald, Board-Certified Nutritionist

The leading cause of mortality in industrialized nations has quickly shifted from infectious diseases prevalent at the beginning of the century to lifestyle and illness related conditions. The majority of standard medical textbooks attribute 50 to 80 percent of all infectious disease to psychosomatic reactions. In other words, to stress. Emotional stress has very real and psychological effects upon a body.

Judith Orloff, M.D.

Love is the highest, most powerful force in the universe, and that to shape one's life, one must believe in the power of love, and if ever you have a doubt about anything, or your lost, or you don't have a direction to go you always follow the power of love. The answer is to always come from the heart. And what is love. Love is the ability to have kindness, and empathy and openness, and a sense of connection with others and with life.

Unconditional love is something that comes from your heart. It literally comes from your heart chakra, or the heart energy center here, that comes as a result of the loving kindness you can show yourself and others. And it's an energy you can develop. Love is an essence of mental health, it's the essence of healing, it's the essence of everything. And one can develop love and unconditional love through power of mediation, through the power of good acts, through the power of feeling energy as it flows through the body. As I do energy healing on people, I call on the power of love to flow through me, to have it do the healing. And it's that healing force of love that has the power to change everything.

Love has the power to change the world. If our political leaders valued that above all else. Above all righteousness, above this god against that god, us versus them, then we would have the power to create some kind of enduring peace, but the thing about knowing the power of love, one must find it through intuition, this isn't just through the mind. One must feel the power of love in oneself and allow that experience to propel yourself and to believe in it, and believe that the power of love is greater than any darkness, greater than any fear, and it's political leaders, social leaders that set that as a priority. Then when they go into these summits, they go into these meetings, they can set that intention to resolve the differences. And not get caught in the tit for tat linear mind interactions that will only create war, because from an intuitive standpoint, there is absolutely no such thing as us versus them. Nothing, it's only we.

Ashok Gangadean, Ph.D., Professor of Philosophy

What is deep love? Deep love is not a feeling, or psychic state of mind. It is the flow and energy of the universe itself. So that whether you're using the tao language or the Buddha language or the Christ language or the Arab language or Allah, the infinite is infinitely connected, in infinite union and communion, and unity and flow, and harmony, and that harmony is love where everything is in this nonviolent flow. If that's love then it's the fabric of reality itself. The essence of being, to use that talk. That in a way if we are in touch by some miracle with that flow of love, which our teachers have called us to do, because when we break out of an ego separated, cut-off form of life, an ego based way of looking at yourself, which disconnects you to an awakened space, letting go of that ego box, and stepping outside into love, and touch reality and interconnectivity to see that beauty in nature in that sunset, to see the beauty in that persons eyes, your beloved's eyes, or the beauty of a child, or in the words of your teacher, whatever it may be. That love is all foundationally interconnected with the interconnected flow of reality. When you touch interconnectivity, you're touching the fabric, the energy of reality itself. And in that flow of communion, that deep love, is really at the heart of all forms of love. So when we hear in our spiritual traditions, that God is love, for example, or to love one another, or to love God is to love one another, and so forth. These are all axioms and theorems of the same principle, that we are love, because the energy of reality is the energy of harmonious communion.

Unconditional love is not the same as ego based love. Ego based relationships, ego based life is disconnected, fragmented, polarized, and Martin Bubler for example, tried to get this vocabulary. So there's a difference between the 'I' it, where the other is an "it," an object, an entity, and I thou, where the other is a person, a mensch, a lover. And yet our society continues to be illiterate on these two dimensions of language, and living, and relating, or not relating. If your living in an ego based 'I' it ego mental life, love in this deeper sense is not available, we're cut off. And yet it calls us in every pulse of our life, because life is love, because in this language we can go into the deeper flow that Jesus understood. He spoke from love, he was love. When he spoke from love he saw the interconnectivity, even with your enemy. Love your enemy. Or the call to our origins of the Judaic tradition. Love God with all your heart, mind and soul. It's a love issue. What is it to love God? To be in the communion of that interconnectivity, which is unconditional love. Conditioned love is ego based love, with conditions. If I get this you get that, you're an object, you objectify one another and yourself and love disintegrates. You can't have your love. So the great teachers understood, Buddha understood, in the principle of interconnectivity, which is called compassion, which is feeling with, compassion with, feeling compassion with, that is love, when you flow in compassion in the zone of reality, you feel you interconnectivity with your other.

Love is opening the space, the sacred space, to encounter

the other, let her, or him, speak in their own voice to you. Then love flows. That's unconditioned love. So when we don't have unconditioned love, and very literate and blocked, and cut off from that, it is a desperate tragic situation to enter into real love.

The question of unconditional love, which is not often understood, or even the topic of love itself is not understood really. Look at the wisdom of our great teachers on the planet. That's a perspective I'm bringing, whether you listen to Jesus, or Buddha, Moses, Abraham, Mohammed, just to name a few. Gandhi, Martin Luther King are wisdom keepers. Through the ages men and women, the greats of cons, who've really given us great insight into the meaning of love. Yet love is still misunderstood. We are almost illiterate in the language of love, because of our ego based dominant culture. It all turns on this, because our teachers, our wisdom teachers understood, that if we're living in an ego mindset, or an ego lens of the mind, where you see yourself as a separate disconnected entity, and a being, then you get disconnected from reality and the flow, which is profoundly interconnected. Reality is a unified infinite feel and flow of energy. Whatever name you give. Whether it's God, Yahweh, Krishna, Yoga, Ohm, emptiness, Allah, energy of nature, whatever word you use for the fundamental reality. It's well known that there's a fundamental unified field of reality where everything is in a flow of interconnectivity. That is the source of love. You call it God, or Yahweh, then it follows as an axiom or a science of the unified field. That God is love. We've heard of that. We don't understand what that means because we use a unified language, that chops up and disconnects from that flow. To me this is the fundamental issue concerning love and unconditional love, and the almost pathetic, tragic attempt of ego based love, and life, and cultures, and people. Disconnected from love.

NO MORE DEPRESSION OR ANXIETY

Robert Thurman, Ph.D.

I teach at Columbia University; it's supposed to be a great university. And we don't teach our students to be decent human beings. The president, during orientation when they arrive and graduation when they leave, maybe mentions something about the word decency, and how you're supposed to be decent, but all they're trained is how to be manipulative, how to be clever, how to trick and outwit people, and how to operate under high stress, divert gratification, race like rats one treadmill to another goal and achieve some new thing, we're talking about the high achiever, and then their supposed to get ahead so they want to go straight out into Wall Street, rush off to some big firm and make more money, and they don't know how to treat their wives, they don't know how to treat their children, if they succeed they have a third trophy wife, four sets of divorced children, it's a mess. They have big money, then they die of a heart attack if they don't have a quadruple bypass, to last a couple more years. This is their life, and this is our fault, the Ivy League, Harvard, you know all these places, the prep schools, and even the high schools. And we are producing these monsters really, who have very unsatisfying lives themselves.

During our child development period, especially in fetal growth from the last half of pregnancy through the first six years of our lives, we learn from our parents, and our family, and community, we learn the characteristics of what life is all about. We download their beliefs and their behaviors into our life and then try to live our life based on those experiences. So that if we come from a situation where the concept of love is not really applied to the child or given to the child in its fullest understanding then the child could only pick up the pieces through developmental programming of what love represents and then search for those pieces and therefore we really have a narrow focus of what we're looking for in love, especially if we have a little checklist of "these are the things I must find, then I will know I'm in love," rather than having a much fuller expansion. The problem is our quest is limited by our programming. So whatever your parents found represented love, this is what you're looking for in love, even though there's probably a much grander scheme that we really want, we will look to fulfill the programming of our beliefs and the programming we received when we were children.

Everyone has compassion to their own kin, to those who identify to their own circle of concern, and of course people should have compassion for themselves, actually some people don't, but most people tend to. Therefore the question becomes, how do you enlarge that circle of compassion to include people who are not your kin to be within your circle of compassion. And this is something that requires cultivation you could say. People could go expand and include the team, they could include the tribe, they could include the town, and maybe the nation. In certain times and moments, but then it doesn't last. And so how do you develop an attitude that all beings deserve compassion that your own child would. And to really have that fully expressed, you have to become enlightened. You have to realize your interrelatedness with all beings, and actually with every animal. The idea that animals have no soul, or that there are just living beings and they're some sort of material mechanism, is rejected in the compassion tradition in Buddhism. The basic gist of the method is to see through one's sense of separateness from the world, and deepen one's sense of openness of the world, and then the suffering of others as intolerable as one's own suffering is the ideal.

Ervin Laszlo

There's prevalence that has been around for a hundred years. And people think it has been around at all times, but that is really not the case. The myth is that the more money you have the happier you are. Now, in the middle ages, even in our western world, in Europe, happiness was not conceived purely in terms of material goods. There were the commercial people, there were merchants, but people who had positions of influence, of status, were not necessarily those who were wealthy. Those who had status were those who had honor, those who can help others around them, who had a position where people can look up to them as people of integrity, people of wisdom. Now, today we think status is connected with money; therefore money is something that buys things. Money is the key to everything including happiness. We permit such people to exist because we assume that because they have money they must be happy. Yet all the research, and everyday evidence shows, that beyond a certain point of material goods, beyond a certain point of financial accumulation, the happiness quotient goes down. People become more stressed, more worried. I know a number of people who are super rich and always concerned with the latest movement in the stock market, or always concerned with their enterprises, and what the competition does. They can never extricate themselves from the rat race as it were. And it doesn't help to have lots of money, lots of goods, because your neighbor might have a little more. They're always in completion with the others. So happiness is not there by simply being able to accumulate your material goods around you. It's much more coming into yourself and recognizing you can fulfill what your really here for. That you can fulfill by giving whatever you are getting. By being part of a community, part of the great rhythms of life, instead of accepting yourself only at your own interest. That doesn't make you happy.

Rabbi Michael Lerner, Ph.D., Editor, Tikkun *magazine*

From the earliest ages we are taught that compromising is

Experts Speak Out

the only way to be realistic in this world, and that you have to abandon what you really believe in, in order to be fitting in to the way things are actually structured in this world. The problem is, the more that we compromise, the more that we abandon the highest thing that we believe in, love, kindness, generosity, caring for others, um celebrating the grandeur and wonder of the universe, having pleasure and joy at being alive, the more that we sacrifice those in order to achieve whatever is achievable in the way our workplace is structured, the way our family life is structured, the way our social order is structured, the more we find ourselves being miserable and unhappy. Screw realism. Don't be realistic. Don't accommodate to the world the way it is. Try to transform the world, and what you find is, that your surrounded by people that will be telling you, oh that's so immature of you, so adolescent, grow up. So one thing I try to tell every group of teenagers I meet is don't grow up, if growing up means accommodating to the existing set of constraints in the social order, the social order that favors money, power, domination and control over others. Instead, hold onto the values of love, of caring for each other, of going for a world that is spiritually and ethically centered, and a life that is spiritually and ethically centered. Do not compromise with that world, and tell your friends, and tell the other people you know, that you don't want to compromise, and you know that they too would want life in a different world.

There's a big disconnect between those values that we hold of compassion and generosity and the actual way we've organized our society, but the truth is most human beings actually desire a world of compassion, a world of generosity, a world of kindness, only they don't think it's possible, only they begin to build fences around themselves, in which they screen out the abilities of being loving and kind and generous on a larger level because they think that it's impossible that they themselves will be the only ones that go for it, so for example there is a tremendous amount of people in the right, the center, and the left who individually engage in acts of caring and generosity. When it comes to the larger sphere they feel that there's absolutely no possibility of changing anything in the larger sphere, so they accept social policies that are very ungenerous. What appears to be insensitivity is what I call surplus powerlessness. That is people making themselves feel more powerless than they actually have to be, but that's because everyone approaches it as if we are an individual alone. Actually what we need is a social movement that collects our capacity to change the world. Let me give you an example. When I pass a homeless person in the street, I immediately ask myself, shouldn't I be bringing this person to the shelter of my home? Then I think about the next person, shouldn't I be bringing that person home to my home, and pretty soon I'm overwhelmed by the thought of, "Oh, wait a second. I don't actually have that much room at my home, and if I have to bring all these people to my home, and what if it turns out that some of them are actually dope dealers, or alcoholics, or that they rip my home off," or whatever. So I begin to feel like, "Oh no." I begin to worry about myself when I should be worrying about them. But it's reasonable to worry about myself, but I don't really want to deal with that on the individual level. I wish there were enough housing for everybody, but there isn't, and society won't build the housing, so I begin to close off. I don't want to be this upset all of the time, I do feel great upsets when I see people in the streets, so I begin to close down, to shut off my capacities at generosity and caring for other people, not because I'm fundamentally ungenerous, but because I see no way that myself can deal with this, in other words I don't want to blame any individual American, I don't want to blame people one by one and say you aren't generous or you aren't caring enough. I do want to say that we need a social movement that can enforce that, can demand it.

Henry Grayson, Ph.D., Author, Mindful Living

I think the time of awakening is coming here, as we are approaching the end of the Mayan age, era, or calendar. We are approaching a time when there can be a dramatic shift in our consciousness, our collective consciousness, our awareness that we are something much more than that empty little person that has to do all these external controlling things and acquiring external things in order to be happy and whole and complete. Once we get past that then there truly could be peace on Earth. I think it's about time, I prefer that to all the wars. How about you?

Men have a lot of difficulty communicating their feelings and their needs, and in so many different ways as well about love and sex with their partner. Our culture has not really been one that's supportive of men expressing what they feel, so often the problem is that men don't even know what they feel. How can they express it if they don't know? So we have a very broad cultural problem going on with how we bring up our boys because that's what prepares them to be able to have intimacy or not have intimacy. If they're brought up not to know what they're feeling, or how to express it when they do know it, how can they begin to express it with their partners. How can they show what they need, when they need to be tough all the time, they need to be independent? How can they say I need something? So we have to let them be permissible to us, even to feel such feelings. Then be able to show them that we aren't losing our masculinity because we're showing our feelings and expressing our needs. So we have a major problem that goes underneath this whole problem of a man with his mate. It's a whole party of how we've developed, and a lot of times we have to work on ourselves to get past all of those conditionings we received when we were kids, and to learn that it's okay to have softer feelings, that it's okay to cry, that it's okay to be vulnerable.

It's okay therefore to show that I have a need or a desire, and unless that part's dealt with, it's going to be hard for that man to communicate that with his mate.

So much of the time we are seeking love, we are seeking a partner to bring us love. We feel so empty inside ourselves without love, we feel like love is a commodity and it lies out there with some other person, like if I go out to the right store I'll find the right item to purchase. And we treat relationships that way. We think that if we find the right person, that treats me the right way, then we will have love in our life. Of course, all that does is make me feel more powerless, and when we get into the relationship, anything that's done that doesn't feel loving from the part of the other person, I feel deprived of love again, because I've forgotten one major factor which is I am love itself. I am my own source. I'm not separate from love. I never could be separate from love. I could not exist if I was separate from love, but as Einstein put, we live in the illusion that we are separate. As long as we're in that illusion of separateness we might seek someone else to complete us, or to make us whole, or expect someone outside us to be the source of love. It's better to remember that I am a force of love every time I'm extending it. It's a reminder to me that I'm love. Because if I'm giving love, how can I be giving something I don't have, and have something I am not. So it's a wonderful reminder when I give it that I have it. It's like that oft quoted prayer by Francis of Assisi, when he said, "It is in giving that we receive." I think that's why that phrase has been quoted by thousands of people throughout the centuries. Because it recognizes a basic truth that who I am is love itself. It's a reminder to me that I am love, and in so doing, then we can pick a partner who is going to be like a wonderful dancing partner with us in life, rather than someone who is going to be the total source of happiness and fulfillment for me. The latter way is just a way of setting up failure, and desperation, and littleness, and then resentment and anger. I prefer the former, where if I can recognize that if I am love itself, anytime I need it I can just extend it towards somebody, and as I do that I'm attracting it back. What better way is there than that.

Christopher Cortman, Ph.D., Author, Your Mind: An Owner's Manual For a Better Life

There's a research study that shows that people who cry live longer than people who don't cry. That's a nice little advantage. There's another research study that says the biochemistry of tears is different, according to what kind of tears they are. If there's a tear falling that's designed to clean debris from your eyes, that has a different biochemical makeup than an emotionally based tear, and an emotionally based tear produces a level of cortisol, which is the stress hormone in the body. So merely by crying emotional tears, I'm reducing my stress level. Some people are so uncomfortable, but as a psychologist, I'll tell you, I love it when people cry, because I know at that point they've nailed it. They've felt exactly what they needed to feel, and this is the point of expressing and release, and I'm seeing healing, because they're letting that go, and we will not have to go back to that point. They've flushed it. It's literally a flushing. Catharsis is the Greek word. And so let's never ever run away from tears, and for the men out there let's keep in mind that you have the same tear ducts that a woman has and you have all the same emotions. It's just that for men we are basically taught what are good things, like humor, expressing of love and emotions, which is limited, and then there's anger. And so, if you feel frightened, you cover it up with anger. If you feel humiliated, you cover it up with anger. If you feel rejected, you cover it up with anger. If you feel insulted, you cover it up with anger. Everything's about anger, because we weren't taught as men, that we can experience and express the full gamut of human emotions. However, a fully functioning human is not unlike a brand new car, where all the parts work. That's how you know a person is fully functioning, because he or she can have a belly laugh. He or she can feel sad or cry. He or she has the capacity to feel guilt when it's appropriate. He or she will feel joy, can see a baby and their face lights up, and can have compassion for an elderly person. That's a fully functioning human. It's not one who's so self protected, because there's not a full investment anywhere. That's not a fully functioning person.

Susan MacNeil, Ph.D., Clinical Psychologist

Intimacy with one's deepest nature, to my mind is the intimacy of the soul. Otherwise, who are we? How do we identify and integrate with the intimacy of our soul. What are the qualities? We know that the qualities are love, peace, and strength, and that intimate relationship with our true self is how then we can have the intimate relationship with others.

Intimacy is vulnerability. When we have intimacy with another we are our true selves, and we are very vulnerable, but vulnerability is strength. And it is so essential when we open ourselves to another and commit ourselves to another. We also have our own identity, we don't lose our identity through this intimacy.

When we have a profound, tender, affection for another person, we can be in danger of losing ourselves in them and then it's not an organic, mature relationship. It can take over our lives in a sense. And then we really don't know who we are. It's about the reflection of the other. It's always important that when we do love the other to see that reflection, and understanding, and see a mirror through ourselves in the other. But not with merging.

Experts Speak Out

Peter Reznik, Ph.D., Integrative Psychotherapist

We come into this world with a purpose. We come to climb the ladder of ourselves, and one of the most challenging and the highest aspect of this climb is being loving, learning how to love. There are different forms of love. Some are easier to execute, and some are easier to practice than others. For example there is the love of a parent. That's relatively easy. If the person is not mentally ill, they will love their child. There is love for your pet. There is love of a student for a teacher. There is love of the teacher from the student. And then there is romantic love, and that gets a little bit more complicated, because there is not only great affection for a person that you love, but also a great desire to enhance a person's well-being, but also the desire to merge with the person, physically.

Can love ever die? Absolutely it can. In many different ways. One, love can be killed. Killed by a shock, by a shock of betrayal. Whether it's somebody not living up to the promise of being protector, when a man gets scared and runs away leaving his woman behind. I'm giving an extreme example, and that shock can kill love, the pain of recognition that the person was betrayed. Or in infidelity love can be suffocated. Yes, it starts as love. Or someone in the relationship becomes too needy, or jealous. And the person who is the recipient of this jealousy is no longer capable to appreciate the other person, but they are in the mode of survival, and if it lasts for a long time love suffocates. Another way of killing love, or making love fade away is when a couple doesn't make an effort of spending time together, they have their separate lives. Yes they fell in love, and then they are too busy with life. Or they have children and it becomes all about the children. They do not invest in the relationship, and love can fade away. It doesn't mean that if love fades away you never loved each other. It was there. But you did not make an effort. You did not nourish that love. And as I said, it's like a baby. In order to grow, mature, and become that real love that which we are all dreaming, you need to make a great investment.

Harold Shinitzky, Psy.D., Author, Your Mind: An Owner's Manual for a Better Life

It's curious when we talk about the phrase sarcasm. Sarcasm is an interesting tool. It can be both funny and hurting. If someone's sarcastic about something in general it can be very funny, very witty, but if you're sarcastic at someone else's expense, that's hurt, that's abuse, that's wrong. When we look at the research in terms of healthy relationships, they talk about often times there five positive comments are made for every one negative comment. An unhealthy relationship, it's one to one. It may feel one to five

We've confused love with need. It might feel one to five, but it's actually here's one positive, but here's a negative. You get these hypercritical loved ones or parents, and they say you did this good, *but* this isn't done. So you're teaching it's never good enough. It's never enough, you can't be right, you're always wrong. And so you're belittled, you're devalued, no matter what you've done, even when you're trying to do something, the desired behavior, it should be reinforced. Instead you've got this hypercritical individual who then starts cutting, and that's where abuse takes place. And so when we look at the healthy relationships we encourage people, we can just focus on your dynamic right there. The normal process.

I tend to also want to encourage families and couples in particular, it's far less important to prove that you're right, than it is for you to get along. Compromise, negotiate, being thoughtful for someone else. Think about it. A loved one expresses to you something that they would like, and if somehow that's an abusive thing, like they say, I'd like you to speak at a lower voice, you don't have to yell. I'll listen to what you have to say. And somehow the person doesn't hear that as, oh wait a second, I can compromise? I don't have to be screaming just because that was the way I was taught. Most people that are abusive come from abusive backgrounds. Just because you come from an abusive background doesn't mean you will become an abusive individual. But if you are, it's usually based on something you've been exposed to. Something that you've seen, it feels normal, you've been role modeled. And for those individuals, getting this type of loving feedback is vital. To be able to develop new skills is a challenge. And for them to be motivated when we look at these stages of change, are they out of place to make this type of committed change, to get someone to compromise, negotiate, communicate, show compassion and be thoughtful. That's vital in a relationship.

A good helper is a good listener. An old saying at that Dr. William Ulcer, at Johns Hopkins, used to say, 'seek to understand and only then will you be understood,' well that was a quote fro, I believe, St. Francis of Assisi. One of the things he took from that is it's far more important to know what person has this disease, then to know what disease this person has. It's amazing to think that there's this human dynamic that we're talking about, where some people run from it. The best providers tap into that connection.

Joyce Hawkes, Ph.D., Biophysicist & Cell Biologist

For me being, coming through hardcore science, I was trained in the cellular end of survival of the fittest. What happens to cells as they evolve into beings and species as they evolve. But my personal experience was discovering the power, if you will, of compassion, and the information that comes out of cultures where cooperation and compassion work, rather than competition. So I see in that sweep of things, the efficacy of compassion. At a cellular level, compassion has now been shown to create neurogenesis. The brain cells in the cortex of our brain that are crucial for cognition for doing all of the mental activity that we do, especially when we age, are replaced when we engage exercise, fine motor skills, and compassion. This is an amazing thing that there's actually cells in our body that respond to the emotion, the actions of compassion. It was said at some time that the minutes that we're born into life, we have all the brain cells we're ever going to have. The truth is, our brain cells do divide and replenish very slowly, and technology has had to develop to be able to show us that they actually do divide, the do reform, and compassion is actually one of the facilitators, a main driver, that allows those brain cells to be replenished. I think that's really incredible news, and allows us to develop what I believe is natural to us as human beings. I see it in animals also. There is a sense of cooperation in many species as there are in humans, and we move and walk in our lives with a true sense of cooperation and acknowledgement, honoring each other. Life certainly goes better in our communities, but it also goes better in our own bodies, inside.

CHAPTER 11

Testimonials

Jacqueline Cox, age 46

Gas was a problem. This has been reduced. Ridges in my nails have disappeared. I have lost weight. The color of my skin has changed and it looks better. I am sleeping more. I am tired at 11:30 at each night and am getting more sleep. I have more regular and daily bowel movements. I had some chest pains. They have reduced and I have only had one episode in the last three months. My skin is not as dry and is softer. My sugar cravings have reduced.

Shawn Cox, age 35

I have lost 15 pounds. I have lost the negative mindset that would stop me from achieving my goals. I can see things that I could not see before that are the most important in my life such as spending time with my family.

Marsha Perry Starkes, age 49

My brain fog is beginning to lift. I am able to see my shortcomings more easily. I am able to develp self-motivation, especially in exercising. I have lost six to seven pounds.

NO MORE DEPRESSION OR ANXIETY

Michael Johnson, age 46

My blood pressure went from 180/110 to 150/90. I have diabetes and my sugar level was averaging 140–160. Now it is 80–140. I lost 10 pounds. I believe I am more forgiving of myself and others.

Andre Partlow, age 26

When I keep my environment clean and uncluttered my thinking is clearer and I just feel better because it's clean and in order. When I don't eat late I sleep deeper, wake with more energy and need less sleep. I also had changes with my blood work.

Yacine Houari, age 51

I had back pain which has improved. I was overweight and I lost 30 pounds. My lack of stamina had improved and I finished the New York City Marathon. My mood has improved and also my skin quality.

Anastasia Koutsouras, age 18

I have lost some weight and body fat. My nails are growing nicely. I don't know if this is related, but my sweat doesn't smell as much. I have mild asthma, but I feel that I can breathe easier now. When I got to bed, I fall asleep right away. I used to toss and turn for a long time before I went to sleep. I've noticed I have more energy.

Lucyna Sadowska

I needed to lose weight and I lost 4 pounds. My concentration improved and also my clarity of thinking and focus. I learned how to control my emotions.

Halina Baranski, age 51

My fatigue is gone. I have better clarity of mind and better completion of tasks. My wrinkles are almost gone.

Tamara Baranski, age 35

Before I was not able to trust myself 100 percent and did not have the will power to quit eggs and cheese. I also had acne. Now I trust myself 200 percent, I have quit eggs and cheese and my acne is almost gone.

Simone Roberts

I came here specifically to lose weight, treat my hypothyroid and my rapid pulse. I am off medication for the hypothyroid and rapid pulse. Instead I took three weeks off from work and feel much better. I am proactive in my medical care, not allowing the doctor to categorize me. The biggest change in me is my mind-set. I have tried for the past three years to be a positive thinker, but with this study it has become a reality. I stop myself from being negative. I also found out I used to be a blamer. Everything is someone else's fault. Now I am working on looking for the positive, what is to be learned and responding in the positive. Thank you all!

Bobby Whitsett, age 45

I notice my skin has more vigor. I notice an increase in strength at the gym. My eyes don't tire as easily and I recall things more. My body fat has decreased and I have more energy to do things after work.

Bridget Carles, age 49

I started the protocol April 15, 2002 in Naples, Florida. I have lost 25 pounds and reversed arthritis in my right ankle and hips. I no longer need a cane. I can power walk one hour each day and can dance, jog, play tennis, and baseball. Formally I barely hobbled around. Many liver age spots have vanished and many have now improved texture and are disappearing. My fatigue is gone. I have three small kids (under 12 years), I work six days and I am never tired anymore. I have a much-improved attitude—joy and positivism. Formerly, I lost all desire for marital intimacy (sex) and hated my husband's requirements. Now my libido is off the charts; my responses are as good or better than 20 years ago. The cells of my body are vibrating in a new, fantastic way.

Tom Graham, age 70

I now have my anger completely under control. I am more spiritual now than I have ever been. I now live in harmony with nature. I exercise now more frequently than I have ever exercised in my life. As a consequence of all these changes, I feel healthier now than ever before.

Francie Smilowitz

During the support group I lost over seven pounds and gained more energy. I have less pain in my body. I created wonderful new relationships which honor the emerging me. Even after I chose a wheat-free diet, I made no effort to set a time to eat. Now I have regular mealtimes and stay on the dietary protocol. I now have better concentration. I took responsibility for each change and chose to honor alignment of mind, body, and spirit so that continually whatever was out of alignment became an awareness to me so I could really make a conscious choice or begin to. I made more time for breath, meditation, and energy work. The weekly reminder of being in the support group where I was present with people who had also chosen to honor and take responsibility for their holistic health, and life was very positive for me. I now take the time to read more, have begun to restructure my relationships, and to express myself more.

Tamarah Cabrera, age 45

My fatigue is gone and I am able to sleep four to five hours a night and feel rested and energized. I have more mental clarity and I can do many things at a time successfully. From being mildly depressed I now am able to look at problem solving in a positive way. Formerly I was doing no exercise at all. Now I am power walking three to five times a week doing yoga three times a week and have participated in races and even the New York City Marathon. I lost 3 percent body fat. Before I participated in the support group I was not able to make decisions. Now I know I can do whatever I would like to and I have the will to follow through!

Harriette Berman, age 58

Previously I had an inferiority complex and confusion of mind; now I have a stronger sense of self and clarity of mind. My depression has lifted and I do not cry so easily. I am better organized and on time. My messiness has lessened. Instead of eating late at night I now eat much earlier. My dry skin has improved, especially my facial skin. I drink much more water now where before I drank none.

Diane Rodriquez, age 50

I have changed my bad eating habits and now eat an organic vegetarian diet. I have much less fatigue but still experience some. I plan to relieve this fatigue by more exercise. I lost 10 pounds. When I was heavier I didn't feel well, couldn't breathe and my upper chest felt heavy. Now I can run and go up stairs easily.

Carol Allen

I had pain in my knees before but now I can do deep knee bends comfortably. I lost eight pounds and have increased the distance of my running. I feel I am just getting started.

Viola Fuentes, age 36

I was afraid and confused. I was overweight and stuck in an unhealthy home situation. The hours stuck in self doubt left me with a fear of being crazy. There was no one to talk to and nowhere to turn. At first I felt, "How could I give up all the food I ate my whole life?" So, I vowed to go on Gary Null's program totally. I lost weight and became a vegetarian. My children and I thrive on the program. I will not ever again tolerate verbal abuse. I set firm boundaries. My children and I recently moved to another state and now we have a peaceful home. Uncluttering the past brought new friends into our lives.

June Bolton, age 56

I always felt tired. I was sick each day and had a chronic walking problem because of hip displacement which fatigued me. I had suffered from various allergies. I was depressed. Exercising several times a week gives me energy and enthusiasm about life. I can do headstands and my body is flexible. I go dancing. I am also 16 pounds lighter and do not have discomfort walking, my allergies improved. My physician is amazed by my younger, youthful body.

Veronica Peters, age 27

I ate junk food and was a heavy coffee drinker. I was hypoglycemic and fainted frequently. My skin had ugly eruptions. I cried easily and had low energy. I had several allergies. I lost 15 pounds. Eventually all my respiratory infections and skin problems disappeared. I still follow the diet and juice during the day, eat fruits in the evening and make one well-planned meal a day. I am now a marathon runner. My energy is without limit. I am healthy.

Cheryl Meer, age 32

I developed severe allergies and upper respiratory infections. I was consumed with family issues which made me angry and anxious. Negative people annoyed me. My past caused me anger. I could not express my feelings or deal with them. I developed a healthier life without colds and other respiratory illnesses. I am now vegetarian. I juice, meditate and see my loved ones with compassion. I understand my anger and anxieties. They are gone. The past no longer plays over and over again in my mind. I actualized a new successful career as a freelance editor; no toxic office environment. I am active in political causes, especially violence against women using hotlines and shelters.

Sara Medeiros, age 36

I had irritable PMS symptoms for 14 years. My sagging skin ages prematurely with pimples, cysts, and scars. My digestive problems caused bloating. Personal relationships were unpleasant. I no longer have PMS problems. My skin is tight and less lined. The pimples and discoloration from cysts are fading. My energy increased. The journals and letter writing self-empowered me. I will take risks with confidence not fear. The new man in my life is far superior to those of my past.

Jozana Smith, age 38

I was overweight and could not slim down. I had acute heartburn, acid reflux, stress, and angry outbursts. Coping with my teenage son was unbelievably stressful. I wanted to change my life and clear my mind. Since following the protocol my body is alive and energetic. I uncluttered my mind and home daily. I handle coworkers and my son without anger. The incredible homework questions made me think as I never did. I am optimistic, more open and accepting, less critical, and patient. I have traded anger for self-love.

NO MORE DEPRESSION OR ANXIETY

Michael Kale, age 44

During my younger years I was involved in drugs, alcohol, ignorance and a complete disregard for others. Rejection was a personal insult, an attack that needed correction. I became angry and sullen and hid myself from actualization. Fear of job loss created a major negative. I was advised to have surgery to remove a pleomorphic adenoma by an ear, nose, and throat doctor. The protocol is a gift of wellness. I am no longer affected by rejection or harbor feelings of diminished self-worth. Liberated of my ego, I became a nicer person at home. I developed spiritually and emotionally. I will continue to follow the protocol and manifest healing of my parotid gland.

Scott Dennison, age 35

I am a construction worker. I felt I was losing stamina and did not know if I could handle my work. I felt my body age. Today I can keep up with younger coworkers; my physical endurance has increased. Injuries and pulled muscles heal quickly. My forgiveness letters allowed me true introspection and I focus on myself, avoiding all toxic situations.

David Michelson, age 47

I began to look and feel middle aged. I was cynical, felt I looked old, dissatisfied with my body, had 13 percent body fat. Was self-critical and drank alcohol. I ate fast foods. These actions stressed me out and seemed to age me. Today I am less self-critical and I do not drink alcohol. I evolved many behavioral adjustments and recently was asked for proof of age to enter a club. That confirmed my success.

Alexandra Mare, age 52

I was dissatisfied with my body. My energy was low and I

was very overweight. My acquaintances and friends were depressing me to the point of irritability. I had a fear of public speaking and did not know where to turn for guidance.

I joined a health support group. Gary Null was informative on the radio, but I could not apply this information in a constructive way.

When I finally did, I lost 16 pounds without dieting. My increasing energy made me feel young again. I need less sleep and find I am not distracted with people people's petty, unimportant issues. I uncluttered my life and am having fewer objects gave me space, a feeling of freedom. My toxic relationships were dismissed, my self-esteem replaced them.

I learned to be the real me, healthy and vital.

Alice Johnson, age 58

I was concerned about my health. My blood pressure and cholesterol were elevated. I had a stressful life and could not control these feelings. I disliked my varicose veins. I suffered with an acid reflux condition that I assumed was caused by my job. My body was falling apart.

I detoxed and carefully followed Gary's protocol. I felt stronger each week and released stress each day. My blood pressure is normal today. My digestion improved, no more acid reflux. I lost 15 pounds. My blood tests are good and my figure it leaner. I am shapelier. I feel cleaner. I do aerobics at home in the morning, yoga during evening hours, and I bike, walk, and run. My uncluttered environment and journal writing give me a new constructive outlook. I use green juices and green and red powders with supplements. My water is pure. I am organic and I am goal-oriented.

Andrea Paredes, age 39

I weighed 300 pounds and wore size 24 or 26 clothing. I was not diagnosed with illnesses but I felt exhausted, had painful varicose veins, back problems, was nauseated after meals, lactose intolerant, and had bad digestion. I ate flesh foods and dairy. I listened to Natural Living and joined a support group.

Today I weigh 225 pounds and wear a size 18. I developed a sense of value in the group and can say "no." I feel centered and empowered. I juice and take supplements. By discovering a new world of health food stores I choose products carefully. As a creative cook, I enjoy translating old recipes into vegan meals using grains. I created a dance area at home and enjoy biking, skiing, kayak class, and swimming lessons.

Damon Keller

I felt frustrated and I could not muster up energy. I overslept, my hair was graying, my sinus infections drove me mad, and my cholesterol and blood pressure were elevated. This was not me, and I had to find a method of true reversal.

I went on Gary's protocol carefully. It was easy. I enjoyed new foods. I learned to understand body mechanisms. My elevated blood levels are normal now. My sinus problems are gone. I sleep less and awake with energy. My hair texture has improved and I have less graying. I am determined to achieve and have relationships with my family.

Ted Jones, age 43

I lost 50 pounds, my body is stronger, my heart is stronger, and my blood pressure is down. I find that my head is clearer. I have not had chronic bronchitis or any colds, and I noticed a recognizable reduction of mucus in nasal passages. I no longer suffer from heartburn. I feel great! I am energetic and happy.

The best part of all of this is that I feel in control of my life. I no longer drink champagne. I've continued the walking program, and I feel my body changing. I've achieved self-esteem, self-reliance, and the notion that I'm the hero in my life. I'm becoming clearer and clearer about how I live my life, and I see how the old ways don't work. I now question why I have certain beliefs. I've reclaimed myself and my life and I am hopeful about my future.

Wanda Bilson

A 20-year-old friend I hadn't seen in a year sees me and says, "Wow! What have you done?" I told him the "Gary Null Thing."

Since starting Gary's protocol, I lost 25 pounds, and went from flab to muscle tone. I am well defined and I get stares in the park now! My joints are limber and I am more flexible, my blood pressure went down 20–30 points, I have more endurance and I can take mental and physical stress better. My digestion has also improved and I have five bowel movements a day. I need less sleep, my hair is much richer, with better texture, and I am viral and horny!

My cognitive functions are also much better, especially my memory. I am less scattered, and calm. I really like running, swimming and power walking. These activities are wonderful and invigorating. It's almost like a spiritual retreat. I have a much greater thirst for spirituality, to find that "something."

Joan O'Keefe, age 23

Gary's support group and protocol helped me battle depression. I gained five pounds, and I now wake up with more energy. I require less sleep and there is noticeably less muscle-lethargy headaches. I feel wonderful.

Kevin Miller

When I began Gary's program I had been putting on some weight. But my big problem was insomnia, insomnia that was caused in large part by medications I was taking for asthma. I was getting two to four hours of sleep a night. Now I am cutting down on some of the medicines, which does help my sleep. However, I think the combination of less medication plus no caffeine, sugar, or wheat in my diet is making the big difference. I am now able to sleep. My other troublesome condition was that I had lost all sense of smell and taste. Now, after four and one-half months, I have both back.

Before joining Gary's program I was feeling lethargic and gaining weight. I have lost 28 pounds and my energy level is much higher. There is a new lightness to my being. I feel great. I no longer have headaches. I can exercise regularly. Everything I do now seems to require much less effort.

Frank Villar, age 29

I am so glad that I joined Gary's support group. Following his protocol, I lost nine pounds, my muscle tone, cardiovascular capacity, and digestion have improved. I require less sleep, my allergies are much better and not clogged up. I meditate after work—it clears my head. Exercise has been the easiest part. After doing my cardio exercise I feel great. I work out at the gym in the mornings and sometimes after work. I walk the golf course instead of riding. Now I trust myself to make decisions and I go with my gut. My home is less cluttered. I have a greater sense of order. I no longer judge or at least am very aware not to judge others. I am now considering moving to a warmer climate. I no longer worry what people think of me. I will not let anyone stop my connection to "my joy." I have disconnected from my negative relationships. My faith is even stronger. The positive voice is beginning to overpower the bad.

Peggy M.

I attended a support group and I was a vegan and longtime

listener of *Natural Living*. I went to Paradise Gardens. Although I felt healthy, I wanted to boost my energy.

The detox gave me incentive to exercise, move my body, but the spiritual and psychological lectures and teachings, although difficult, changed my life. The connection between spiritual health and physical healing is crucial. My quiet moments meditating and using breath work helped me lose seven pounds without dieting, additionally the yoga and exercise builds my muscles.

Raising three children, teaching religion in class and taking yoga lessons create a hectic day. I juice, use green powders and cook healthy vegetarian food. With supplements and diet, I feel well grounded. My vegan meals contain tofu, beans, seeds and nuts, no dairy. Although my husband and children are not totally vegan yet, I still am. I am confident with my priorities. "The quiet moments let us know who we really are, the health follows."

Fran S., age 51

I was motivated towards life changes by listening to Gary on the radio. He was the only person on the air who explained organics, nutrition and the negative impact of substances used by the food industry. This was new, important information and I accumulated facts during each show.

As I made lifestyle changes and became aware of food after it enters the body, I felt and looked healthier. This intensified during my stay at Paradise Gardens where everyone was beginning their actualization. I was impressed to see Gary doing everything he taught. I learned to power walk. Memories of Naples are happy and positive.

Today, I make healthy choices. The dos and don'ts were explained during lectures and in Florida, the protocol is simple and pure. I observe life choices and see various components to health. Choosing a spiritual path begins new processes. I study energetic healing and Natural Force Healing. I chose life and honor the spirit.

Sallie W.

This has been a journey filled with new insights, struggles, changes in lifestyle and eating and enlightening. I have learned much, let go of bad baggage and am still in the process of reclaiming total health and wellness. I am also learning how not to be a victim of what other people choose to do. I have learned not to take things personally and am reevaluating all of my relationships. I have added fun to my life with roller skating and increasing more in daily exercise and diet.

I am making progress that I am proud of. I feel good about myself and growing stronger in areas where I am weak.

After being a frequent marijuana user, my mind is clearing much faster than most because of the protocol. Also, since being on the protocol, my hay fever, which was very severe, causing constant runny nose, repeated violent sneezing, red watery eyes, and congestion so bad I had to breathe through my mouth is GONE! Now I can run like the wind. I joined the cross country team and today I ran five miles.

Maria

At the beginning of the program, I was very tired all of the time. It was difficult for me to get up in the morning. I was tired all day long. My skin had a dark sickly look to it. I had dark circles under my eyes and my skin would always break out with pimples. My hair was falling out. My body was very thin and I had no muscle tone. I have integrated exercise by getting a membership to the YMCA. I also go for walks and ride my bicycle. I have also begun to play the drums in a rock band and have found it to be a fun way to get a great workout.

My skin is now much clearer and healthier looking. My body has more muscle tone now that I work out regularly. I also haven't had a cold in the six months of this program. My nose used to be clogged all of the time but now it is always clear. I have also had my mercury fillings taken out which has resulted in a dramatic increase in energy.

I have a more positive outlook on life than I used to. I still fall into negative slumps sometimes but I am more aware of them so I can get myself out of them.

I had a job that I absolutely hated. It was a "go nowhere" job in an office in a field that I had no interest in. Luckily for me, I was laid off, which has given me a lot of time to focus on music. My band has been traveling and playing shows with such a great response every place we play. This has given me a sense of satisfaction to be able to do what I love to do.

I am a much more happy person spiritually now than ever before. I only surround myself with warm loving nurturing people and I stay away from negative energy. I used to feel that my best days were behind me, but now I feel that they're way ahead of me.

Miranda

Since working with Gary, I generally feel better about me. I really have a better attitude. I lost five pounds, my energy level is higher, and I feel more alert and rested in the mornings. My cravings for sweets diminished, my ingrown toenails healed and my scalp dryness eased. I've become more open and confident.

Hyacinth

Growing up I was taught that there is only one way to be healthy: by eating the correct foods. However, on joining the program, I've learned so much about how the body works and is nourished by other nutrients and the process the body goes through.

My belief was not quite correct. It was a challenge to change my lifestyle, but mentally I know it was the right change. I was always ready to help anyone who wanted to make this change in their life, and reaching out to others made me feel good, with some satisfaction. I am focused in my thinking and usually set a goal in my mind and really go after it to allow it to happen. The effect of what was told to me in the program made a complete change in my life, and I am able to rationalize problems in the way of health, not any major one, and conquer the problem.

Today I am a better person in shape as I feel much healthier than before. Many of the nutrients I took, the juices, and the habit of eating organic vegetables, grains, and fruits gave me phenomenal results. My hair is not as gray as before. Patches have come out with the original black renewed hair; my skin is supple, firm, and younger looking. My nails are soft and pink. The arthritis in my fingers diminished, and I don't have those dizzy spells as before.

It's my belief that my cholesterol is much lower. I have lost 17 pounds. I still have to do more in the line of exercises, but this is due to an ailment in the leg. My outlook of appearance is much more appealing to others, as they tell me I look younger. I feel great internally and externally. This physical change is of great importance to me as my health is my happiness. I can do much more at home, as I have more energy. I sleep two hours less and I do not feel fatigued as before. At times, I would feel sloppy on the job, but after attending the classes, I am more alert, think clearly, and am always energetic.

I conquer negative emotions by having a passion for what I want. Being here I am more connected with the Higher being. My prayer life is meaningful to me and others. I share my time with others in their grief and pain, and I can always refer to an encyclopedia, my magnets, and communication with Him. He is always there for me when I need Him. I feel that innermost relationship spiritually.

Behavioral patterns have changed, as I do not have any hatred in my heart for people anymore. It does not get me anywhere when I can change the negativity to something positive by assisting and giving myself in a situation. It is my belief that whenever you can do a good deed or say a good word to someone or of them, it is the correct way in mind and body. I am more spiritually connected and my life is more meaningful of a happier, prayerful life. After taking the green juices, red stuff, and nutrients, I do not have the breathing problem, so I believe my cholesterol has dropped somewhat.

My sister got over her asthma after forty years of her life. She was always in the hospital emergency, and at one time the family thought we would lose her, but she feels great now. I feel much healthier and I feel I'm living a much more meaningful life. This change was with results and I intend to keep on it all my life. I see there is a way of life taking good foods and with supplements and exercise, one has to be on the way to good health.

Liz

I am choosing relationships that are positive.

In the six months since beginning the program, I have changed physically, losing 20 pounds and working out four to five days a week. I have incredible energy and am not tired. I sleep less, but the sleep I get is restful.

Mentally, I am more clear-thinking, making decisions regarding my life and business quicker, as opposed to laboring over them. I have no depression, but a general feeling of grounding and balance. Affirmations work.

I love work! I own my own business, an organic vegan home delivery service. Since being a member of the group, I am more organized—no procrastination. Our company has tripled its business. The company has become an extension of my being.

I have much more quality play in my life, and I choose very carefully who I'd like to play with. My time is important. Most important, because work is demanding, I truly enjoy my "playtime." As far as relationships go, once again, time is valuable, which made it easy to shed relationships that were toxic and draining. I moved out of a six-and-a-half year relationship to a studio apartment that belongs to me-serene, peaceful, and beautiful. I am choosing relationships that are positive.

Although not every day moves gracefully through my life, each day is growing more enjoyable and fun. This support group has helped change my life to a positive, peaceful state of being.

• CONCLUSION •

Let's reflect upon what we've learned. Depression cannot be as easily defined as we've been led to believe. Crises arise in life—losses, fears, insecurities, anticipations, grief—and these can alter our mood. Psychiatry has taken it upon itself to determine that anything that varies from a happy frame of mind can fall into the net of depression. Clearly, there are some people with specific brain chemical imbalances. For those individuals, there are natural and nontoxic remedies that work equally as well but without the side effects of the selective serotonin reuptake inhibitors and other drugs. The vast majority, however, do not fit into this category. Children and seniors, the most vulnerable members of our society, must take special care to stay away from psychiatric manipulation and mass marketing.

Where anxiety and depression do exist, Americans need to pay attention to diet. We eat fast foods—a mind numbing variety of junk foods, foods laced with colorings and pesticides, and now genetically altered foods. We know that sugars, artificial sweeteners, and allergic molecules of food can trigger brain reactions that manifest as anxiety and depression. Add to that the harmful chemicals we breathe and polluted water we drink and you will get an even larger picture of the problem. We live in a toxic cesspool, and this can adversely affect both body and mind. The degree of contamination is so great, in fact, that scientists have correlated its effects to changes in the DNA of unborn children!

Sadly, we are not being honest about the true causes of our dilemma. To do so would be to reveal the corporatization of American culture, where what is good for big business is good for America. Our reaction is, in effect, rather schizophrenic. On one hand we have the Surgeon General, the U.S. Public Health Service, and the National Institutes of Mental Health coming forward and stating that we should clean up our act by taking fast food operations out of hospitals and schools and replacing them with better quality fare. We will not act on this common sense advice, though, because it would mean eviscerating a $300 billion a year industry. Special interest groups contribute substantial amounts of money and, with it, gain access and influence to politicians.

At the end of the day, truth is not what we're given but manufactured—carefully spun propaganda. We're caught in this paradox. We know the truth but cannot utter it. There are too many people who paid for the lie. When you look at the amount of people who have invested in the disease-producing businesses that give us obesity, heart disease, cancer, arthritis, as well as mood-altering illnesses, you see that they are the most powerful among us. They are not the fortune 500 companies, but they have an interlocking board of directors on banks. They include large regimens of scientists, physicians, paid consultants who do their bidding before Congressional hearings and for the major media.

How then does the average person with access to none of the above find the truth and make changes? First, do not wait for the mainstream media. They are, by default, limited in what they can offer. Only the most naïve would still believe that we have a truly free and democratic press. Nor can we count upon the objectivity, reasonableness, and humanity of the medical community. They are too conditioned in their own behavior. We must therefore take it upon ourselves to begin the process of networking, to find health support groups, to find counselors and holistic physicians who can help us identify what may be causing our problems, and who can show us sensible ways of eliminating our conditions and rebalance ourselves.

Millions of Americans are on their own unique journeys of healing. They are moving away from the strictly orthodox point of view and opening themselves up to alternative perspectives. The rest of us would be wise to follow their examples. For further information, go to www.garynull.com; look under mental health and visit our online support group for depression and anxiety.

• APPENDIX •

For Alternative Health Studies

Acupuncture and Eletroacupuncture

At Beijing Medical University, two consecutive clinical studies on the treatment of depression with electroacupuncture (EA) were conducted. Results from both studies showed that the therapeutic efficacy of EA was equal to that of amitriptyline for depressive disorders. EA had a better therapeutic effect for anxiety somatization and cognitive process disturbance of depressed patients than amitriptyline, and the side effects were much less.

In Germany, results indicate that needle acupuncture led to a significant clinical improvement as well as to a remarkable reduction in anxiety symptoms in patients with minor depression or generalized anxiety disorders.

In Minneapolis, alcohol use was assessed, along with depression and anxiety, when treated with acupuncture, and significant improvement was shown on nearly all measures.

In Ontario, Canada, acupuncture was shown to alleviate depression in patients receiving opiates for chronic nonmalignant pain.

At the University of Exeter, acupuncture was shown to be useful in reducing anxiety in the treatment of cancer patients.

At Stanford University, in a review of the efficacy of

selected alternative treatments for unipolar depression, acupuncture was shown to be an effective alternative monotherapy for major depression.

A survey conducted in Padua, Italy, found that acupuncture, among other alternative therapies, had a complementary role for the elderly with depressive symptoms.

In a survey of complementary and alternative medicine (CAM) treatments, the University of Exeter found acupuncture for anxiety useful to cancer patients.

Amino Acids and Tryptophan

Amino acids are building blocks of protein molecules and play a role in the production of mood-regulating brain neurotransmitters. The most important one is tryptophan (L-TP), a precursor to serotonin. But don't be fooled into thinking that just by eating a high protein diet you will get enough tryptophan, and therefore enough serotonin. In order for tryptophan to reach the brain and be converted into serotonin, it must first attach itself onto a certain carrier molecule. Protein meals supply the body with several amino acids, not just tryptophan. And all of these amino acids are competing for a ride on the same carrier. Unfortunately, tryptophan is the least abundant of the amino acids and gets pushed aside by other amino acids, which bully their way onto the transport molecule. As a result, high-protein meals cause both tryptophan and serotonin levels to decline. On the other hand, complete carbohydrate meals, which don't contain tryptophan, are capable of producing a rapid and considerable increase in serotonin levels. Or meals with both protein and carbohydrates also raise serotonin. Turkey is high in tryptophan, just think of all the napping and dozing that goes on after a high-protein, high-carbohydrate, Thanksgiving dinner. Carbohydrates perform this transport function by stimulating the release of insulin. Insulin increases the ratio of available tryptophan, making the carrier molecule more accessible and causing tryptophan uptake.

The amino acid tryptophan is the precursor to serotonin and was used in the 1980s as a treatment for mild to moderate depression. It was in direct competition with Prozac, which was released in 1987. But then in 1989 tryptophan was pulled from the market because it was thought to be the cause of Eosiniphilia myalgia syndrome, which in the United States caused thirty-seven deaths and left over 5,000 permanently disabled. It wasn't long before the real culprit was found, a new genetically-engineered binder added to a tryptophan formulation by a Japanese company. Over $2 billion has been paid in damages by the Japanese manufacturing company. However, tryptophan is still blamed as the cause of the Eosiniphilia myalgia outbreak and has been unavailable to the public ever since. Even though tryptophan is no longer available 5-hydroxytryptophan (5-HTP), derived from a natural plant source (griffonia simplicifolia), is found in health stores. Tryptophan is the direct precursor to 5-HTP which is immediately converted to serotonin. Doses of 50–100 milligrams three times a day can boost brain serotonin levels enough to improve mood, calm anxiety, diminish compulsive behavior, reduce PMS, suppress appetite, decrease carbohydrate craving, improve sleep, and relieve headaches and improve symptoms of fibromyalgia. These are all the things that serotonin is supposed to do naturally, if we give it the right building blocks. The manufacturers of SSRIs don't want you to know this.

In 1978 Acta Psychiatric Scand published a study that claimed 5-HTP did not have an antidepressant effect, and that L-TP, did not appear to be a well documented antidepressant. However this study has been superceded by more recent studies positive for L-TP.

A study in Vancouver found that rapid tryptophan

depletion appears to reverse the antidepressant effect of bright light therapy in patients with seasonal affective disorder.

A study in the United Arab Emirates found that a multiple regression analysis showed a correlation between low tryptophan and increased chance of Edinburgh postnatal depression (EPDS) on day seven after delivery.

After a number of studies challenged the findings that acute tryptophan depletion (TD) increases depressive symptoms in the medicated, formerly depressed patients, a study in Boston found that the mood effect of TD in medicated, formerly depressed patients was confirmed. It suggested a threshold may exists for mood effects following TD, implying that recent negative findings may have been caused by insufficient depletion.

Another study in the Netherlands demonstrated that repeated moderate TRP depletion leads to anxiogenic and depressive-like behavior in the rat and corroborates the notion of the involvement of serotonin in these behaviors.

Alterations in brain tryptophan levels cause changes in brain serotonin synthesis, and this has been used to study the implication of altered serotonin levels in humans. A study in Canada showed that, overall, studies manipulating tryptophan levels support the idea that low serotonin can predispose subjects to mood and impulse control disorders, and higher levels of serotonin may help to promote more constructive social interactions by decreasing aggression and increasing dominance.

Tyrosine is another amino acid that is precursor to an important neurotransmitter, DOPA. It is also a precursor to adrenaline, thyroid hormones, and estrogen. Studies have shown that it lowers blood pressure, suppresses appetite and increases sex drive. But, because it is a precursor to adrenaline it could make a manic episode worse so it should not be used for treatment of manic depression. The average dose is 500mg three times a day. Some feel that more should not be taken without the advice of a health care practitioner. Too much tyrosine may trigger migraine headaches.

Phenylalanine is the amino acid precursor to tyrosine and has been used to treat depression. It should not be used, however, by people who have phenylketonuria (PKU), a genetic disorder that makes it impossible for the body to break down phenylalanine. PKU is usually diagnosed at birth and since a mother does not know if her child could have PKU. Phenylalanine supplements should be avoided in pregnancy. The dosage for phenylalanine is 500mg a day.

Phophatidylserine is an amino acid which works through the hypothalamus to regulate the amount of cortisone produced by the adrenals. Stressful events cause an increase in cortisone in the blood stream, which can keep people on the edge and can lead to depression. Phosphatidylserine helps support and restores nerve cells, and numerous studies show that it slows or reverses cognitive losses attributed to aging.

An article in the *Alternative Medical Review* presents a survey of nutrients and botanicals in the integrative management of cognitive dysfunction and found that phophatidylserine improved mood in middle-aged and elderly subjects with dementia or age-related cognitive decline.

Aromatherapy

Aromatherapy, as one of our studies shows, is a burgeoning new healing modality used by nurses. Concentrated oils from plants are rubbed into the skin for a variety of complaints. These oils contain powerful antioxidants that are absorbed through the skin into the blood stream and can have medicinal effects on the body. The following studies show that certain oils can have a profound effect on anxiety and mood.

The University of Southampton determined that Lavender oil administered in an aroma stream showed modest efficacy

Appendix for Alternative Health Studies

in the treatment of agitated behavior in patients with severe dementia.

In a study at a hospital in Reading, England, patients who received aromatherapy reported significantly greater improvement in their mood and perceived levels of anxiety.

A study in England demonstrated that aromatherapy can be effective in reducing maternal anxiety, fear, and/or pain during labor.

A survey in Seattle, Washington, found that aromatherapy is the fastest growing of all complementary therapies among nurses in the United States.

A study in California found that antioxidants such as eugenol and maltol play an important role in the pharmaceutical activities of natural plant extracts used for aromatherapy.

Ayurveda

Individual herbs and herbal formulas used in Ayurveda, the classical system of Indian medicine, have proven successful in the treatment for depression. For example, a study in Varanasi, India, showed that bioactive glycowithanolides (WSG), isolated from the roots of Withania somnifera, induced an anxiolytic effect, comparable to that produced by lorazepam, in rats. WSG also exhibited an antidepressant effect comparable with that induced by imipramine, in the forced swim-induced "behavioral despair" and "learned helplessness" tests in the rats.

Another study in Varanasi, India, showed that Ayurveda herbal formulation Siotone (ST) reversed the chronic stress-induced increase in rat brain tribulin activity, demonstrating attributes similar to the modern concept of adaptogenic agents which are best known to afford protection of the human physiological system against diverse stressors.

Significant anti-anxiety effects were induced in rats by

low doses of the leaf extract of Azadirachta indica that were comparable to those induced by diazepam.

Bach Flower Remedies

In a survey conducted in the United Kingdom of CAM-providers representing twelve therapies, it was deemed that stress/anxiety was the most common condition alleviated.

Balneotherapy

Balneotherapy is a general term for water-based treatments using natural spring, mineral or seawater to encourage relaxation, improve the circulation, stimulate the immune system, and revitalize and detoxify the body.

Even simple actions such as foot-bathing for 10 minutes in hot water, with or without the addition of essential oil or lavender, can produce beneficial effects. For example, researchers in Japan found the foot-bath produced a significant increase of blood flow. And in the case of a foot-bath with the addition of essential oil of lavender, there were delayed changes to the balance of autonomic activity in the direction associated with relaxation.

Italians found a statistically significant reduction in anxiety and somatisation parameters with arsenic-iron bath treatment for subjects suffering from endogenous reactive anxiety syndromes with somatisation.

A study in Turkey showed that balneotherapy is effective in treating the pain and anxiety of fibromyalgia patients.

In Spain, researchers found that sadness as a feeling of disproportional affective reaction with mental consequences can find relief in spa cures, or balneotherapy.

Bibliotherapy

Bibliotherapy in the form of self-help books, self-help internet sites, or printed material from health-care professionals goes a long way to helping people deal with their feelings of anxiety, stress, and depression.

At the University of Pennsylvania the importance of minimal therapist contact by patients when coupled with mutual-based bibliotherapy interventions (such as self-help books, electronic database searches, correspondence with authors and limited handsearching)led to significant reductions on measures of frequency of panic attacks, panic cognitions, anticipatory anxiety, and depression.

Researchers in Australia found that web sites are a practical and promising means of delivering cognitive behavioral interventions for preventing depression and anxiety to the general public.

Less contact with therapists proves beneficial if patients are supported in learning skills to manage their symptoms (assisted bibliotherapy) from moderate anxiety disorders.

Behavioral problems in children are quite common and many approaches such as medication are limited due to factors such as time and expense. In the U.K. it was found that media-based interventions (bibliotherapy) had both clinical and economic advantages, including the treatment of children with behavioral problems.

Other studies show a wide range of alternatives to counter the negative side effects of conventional medication treatments for depression. For example, calcium is the most abundant mineral in the body. It has profound effects on the nervous system and mood.

Calcium

In Rhode Island a study reported that calcium was effective in reducing emotional, behavioral, and physical premenstrual symptoms.

In New York City, oral calcium supplementation reversed

the reduced vitamin B12 absorption that metformin induced in patients with depression.

Cholesterol

Despite the fact that most people are worried about having cholesterol levels that are too high, yet another study has found that low cholesterol is actually associated with adverse behavioral effects such as aggression and depression.

Cognitive-Behavioral Therapy

Cognitive-behavioral therapy (CBT) is the most thoroughly studied non-pharmacological approach to the treatment of social anxiety disorder, and its efficacy has been demonstrated in a large number of investigations.

At Stanford University, CBT was shown to result in statistically significant reductions of performance anxiety in musicians whereas buspirone was not an effective treatment.

Another study in California of generalized anxiety disorder (GAD) recommended that clinicians should consider the potential benefits of psychotherapy as an adjunct to medication.

Researchers in Albany found that patients showed significant improvements in the quality of life scores after the completion of cognitive-behavioral group therapy for social phobia.

In Rhode Island, a study showed that the efficacy of cognitive therapy in the treatment of premenstrual syndrome.

However CBT, along with other verbal psychosocial treatments for anxiety disorders, has declined in use since the nineties.

A study reported in the *Journal of Psychopathology* recommended that color therapy could be used to follow changes in the state of depressive patients and to predict their response to anti-depressant pharmacotherapy.

In the Netherlands, a study indicated that the colors of antidepressant drugs affected the perceived action of the drug and seemed to influence the effectiveness of the drug.

In Seattle, a computer program (Computer Assisted Relaxation Learning) for conducting exposure therapy for the treatment of dental injection fear, which trained subjects to use physical and cognitive relaxation techniques, was found to reduce their general fear of dental injections.

DHEA

Standard replacement for adrenal insufficiency consists of glucocorticoids and mineralocorticoids while dehydroepiandrosterone (DHEA) deficiency is routinely ignored. However, in Germany, a study demonstrated that DHEA treatment significantly improved overall well being as well as scores for depression, anxiety and their physical correlates in women with adrenal insufficiency. A survey conducted in U.L.B. found that DHEA supplementation has proven beneficial in typical deficient states like adrenal insufficiency or major depressive illnesses.

A study reported in the *American Journal of Psychiatry* found that elevated cortisol-DHEA ratios may be a state marker of depressive illnesses or may contribute to the associated deficits in learning and memory. It recommended that administration of DHEA may reduce neurocognitive deficits in major depression.

At the University of Cambridge, a study found that increased negative mood and feelings as well as DHEA hypersecretion at entry, were associated with subsequent first-episode major depression in adolescents.

In Japan the data in a study suggested a possibility that endogenous DHEA sulphate and dietary soy may modulate psychologic well-being in peri- and postmenopausal women.

Another study at the University of Cambridge

demonstrated that lower DHEA levels are an additional marker for a state of abnormality in adult depression.

At the University of Pittsburgh a study suggested that the decrease in DHEA and DHEA-S remitters is related to remission of depression rather than to direct drug effects on steroids.

Because of the recent large quantities of DHEA sold in health food stores, a team at the University of Cambridge undertook a thorough investigation of well-conducted studies if DHEA supplementation. They support for the claimed improvement in a sense of well-being following DHEA treatment.

Diet

The body is built from what we eat, drink, and breathe. If we choose the healthiest foods and drinks, we have a better chance of building a healthy body. If we choose synthetic, processed foods we increase our chances of ill health because those foods are mostly devoid of nutrients. Vitamins and minerals from healthy food sources provide the healthy co-factors required by all the enzymes in the body. Enzymes run metabolic processes including essential neurotransmitter production and function in the brain. Without proper building blocks and nutrients, these neurotransmitters malfunction resulting in mood and behavioral problems.

In Seattle a study demonstrated that psychological distress is associated with unhealthy dietary practices.

In the U.K. researchers found that the presence of depression was the most powerful predictor of level of well-being, but the finding of a high body mass index is likely to indicate adequate well-being of older people.

In Germany a study showed that dietary treatment cannot be neglected as a possible access to treating hyperactive/disruptive children and merits further investigation.

A series of studies in Norway suggested a correlation

between somatic and neuropsychiatric symptoms and emotional disturbances, and they noted that patients identifying themselves as sensitive to food and chemicals had higher scores for depression, anxiety, shyness, and defensiveness.

A survey in the U.K. revealed that certain dietary risk factors for physical ill health are also risk factors for depression and cognitive impairment. For example, cognitive impairment is associated with atherosclerosis, type 2 diabetes and hypertension, and findings from a broad range of studies showed significant relationships between cognitive function and intakes of various nutrients, including long-chain polyunsaturated fatty acids, anti-oxidant vitamins, and folate and vitamin B12.

A review summarizing the most important research, particularly that from 1985 to 1995, on the relationship between diet and behavior concluded that diet definitely affects some children. Symptoms which changed included those seen in attention deficit disorder (ADD) and attention deficit hyperactivity disorder (ADHD), sleep problems, physical symptoms, with later research emphasizing particular changes in mood.

Drumming

Drumming is a recent therapeutic technique which comes to us from aboriginal cultures. A study conducted in Pennsylvania found that group drumming music therapy is a complex composite intervention with the potential to modulate specific neuroendocrine and neuroimmune parameters in a direction opposite to that expected with the classic stress response.

Essential Fatty Acids

Essential Fatty Acids (EFAs) are also called vitamin F,

designating the nutritional aspects of fats and oils. Essential means that we all need certain amounts of these fats for optimum health. EFAs maintain and enhance normal brain development and functioning. EFAs are also building blocks for hormone-like substance called prostaglandins that regulate immune system functions and play a central role in stress reduction.

There are two main essential fatty acids: omega-3 fatty acids and omega-6 fatty acids. Omega-3 fatty acids are also called alpha linoleic acids found in flax and hemp oils. Omega-6 fatty acids are called linoleic acids found in flax, hemp, borage, and evening primrose oils. Other nonessential but healthy oils are: eicosapentaenoic acid (RPA) found in fish oil; and gamma linolenic acid (GLA) found in borage, hemp, and plentiful in evening primrose oil.

An article in the *Journal of Reproductive Medicine* reports that three studies all demonstrated that evening primrose oil is a highly effective treatment for the depression and irritability associated with premenstrual syndrome.

A study in Boston found that omega-3 fatty acids were well tolerated and improved the short-term course of illness in patients with bipolar disorder.

An article in *Biological Psychiatry* reports that a study showed that three behaviorally different mental disorders were ameliorated with supplements of a newly discovered trace omega-3 essential fatty acid (w3-EFA).

A team in Japan previously found that DHA intake prevented aggression enhancement at times of mental stress. In this study they investigated changes in aggression under nonstressful conditions and found that aggression levels remained stable in the DHA group.

Exercise

From the runner's high, which stimulates a rush of adrenaline, to the calming effects of a walk through the woods, exercise has the power to lift one's spirits.

A survey in Norway found beneficial psychological effects of exercise are best documented for mild to moderate forms of unipolar depression, and in panic and generalized anxiety disorders. It is suggested a simple and inexpensive approach like exercise is helpful and might be important for public health.

In an Australian survey for complementary and self-help treatments for depression, exercise was cited as one of several as having the best evidence of effectiveness.

In California a study found that a twelve-step exercise program for women who were caring for relatives with dementia increased knowledge of the benefits of exercise, increased motivational readiness for exercise, and alleviated perceived stress, burden and depression. The study demonstrated the feasibility and success of delivering home-based health promotion counseling for improving physical activity levels in a highly stressed and burdened population.

Flavonoids

Bioflavonoids, or flavonoids, are plant pigments found in all plants.

The data collected in a paper in Argentina makes clear that some natural flavonoids are CNS-active molecules and that the chemical modification of the flavones nucleus dramatically increases their anxiolytic potency—in one case creating a drug 30 times more potent than diazepam.

Another study in Argentina found that Tilia species, traditional medicinal plants widely used in Latin America as sedatives and tranquilizers, extracted in a complex fraction containing as yet unidentified constituents probably of a flavonoid nature, when administered in mice, had a clear anxiolytic effect but no effect on total and ambulatory locomotor activity.

In Germany a study found that the antidepressant effect that apocynum leaves on male rats in a forced swimming test indicated antidepressant activity comparable to the tricyclc antidepressant imipramine. It further speculated that this effect might be related to hyperoside and isoquercitrin, which are major flavonoids in the extract.

Folic Acid

Folic acid is a member of the vitamin B family and is well known for its ability to prevent birth defects in infants when taken during pregnancy. An article in the *Townsend Letter for Doctors and Patients* reported on a study whose results indicated that supplementation with folic acid may increase the efficacy and reduce side effects of fluxetine in women with depression. Patients with depression have consistently been found to have low plasma and RBC folate levels, and low plasma folate has been associated with a poor response to antidepressant medications.

Guided Imagery

Guided imagery refers to a number of techniques including simple visualization or a direct suggestion. The mental image formed in a guided imagery session may be seen, heard, tasted, smelled, touched, or felt. Therapeutic guided imagery allows patients to experience a relaxed state of mind and then focus on images associated with their problems. A dialogue is then created with their problem out of which often come answers and understanding. Or, simple visualization can take one on a relaxing journey to a safe place in nature and help diminish stress.

The Holistic Nursing Practitioner reported on a study that found subjects who listened to a guided imagery/relaxation tape before their magnetic resonance imaging (MRI) scan had lower levels of anxiety and moved less during the MRI scan.

A study in Louisiana revealed that surgical patients listening to Relaxation with Guided Imagery (RGI) audiotapes demonstrated significantly less state anxiety, lower cortisol levels one day following surgery, and less surgical wound erythema.

In Kansas a study found that guided imagery lowered the anxiety levels of nursing students learning to perform their first injections and recommended introduction of this teaching strategy early in the curriculum.

Researchers in Philadelphia found that guided imagery was well received by bereaved spouses with promising psychoimmunological trends that merited more rigorous investigation.

A study in Miami showed that guided imagery and music (GIM), when used on healthy adults, resulted in significant decreases between pre-and post-session depression, fatigue, and total mood disturbance, and had significant decreases in cortisol level by follow-up. It suggested such changes in hormonal regulation may have health implications for chronically stressed people.

An article in the Journal of Holistic Nursing reports how guided imagery protocol applied to the first 4 weeks of the postpartum period resulted in less anxiety and depression and greater self-esteem in primiparas.

The Annual Review of Nursing published a review of 46 studies regarding the use of guided imagery in the management of stress, anxiety, and depression published between 1966 and 1998 which pointed to preliminary evidence of its effectiveness.

A study at the Group/Walther Cancer Institute explored the effectiveness of guided imagery in alleviating mood disturbance and improving quality of life in cancer patients. The results indicated it significantly improved mood and quality of life in these cancer patients.

A study published in the *Journal of Gerontology Nursing*

indicated that discharge teaching using guided imagery has the potential to decrease depression in older adults after discharge from the hospital.

Herbs

Herbal medicine has a much larger role in Europe in the treatment of mood disorders than in the United States. The most important mood-enhancing herb is St. John's wort. It has antidepressant, anti-anxiety, and sedative properties as well as being a strong anti-inflammatory. Research indicates that its antidepressant effects are due to its serotonin reuptake inhibition properties, which keep serotonin levels elevated. This is the same mechanism by which Prozac works, but without the side effects.

Many other herbs are effective in treating depression and anxiety. In Germany one study showed that a unique extract of black cohosh is associated with improvement in menopausal symptoms, including mood changes, without evidence of estrogen-like effects.

A study in India reports that ginkgolic acid conjugates (GAC) isolated from the leaves of Indian Ginkgo biloba showed consistent and significant anxiolytic activity in rats.

A team in Ottawa, Canada, found that Gotu Kola attenuated the peak acoustic startle response (ASR) in healthy human subjects after earlier studies showed that Gotu Kola decreased locomotor activity and attenuated ASR in rats.

Researchers in Germany did a study that confirmed the anxiolytic efficacy and good tolerance kava-kava special extract WS1490.

A study at the Duke University Medical Center suggested that kava-kava might exert a favorable effect on reflex vagal control of heart rate in generalized anxiety disorder patients.

A study in London demonstrated that kava-kava relieved

Appendix for Alternative Health Studies

total stress severity as well as stress-induced insomnia.

Also in the U.K., an extensive review of published and unpublished studies of Kava-kava extract implied it is superior to placebo and relatively safe as a symptomatic treatment for anxiety.

In Germany researchers found that Kava pyrones exhibit a profile of cellular actions that show a large overlap with several mood stabilizers, especially lamotrigine.

A study in Basel found that there were no residual sedative effects (hangover) the morning after ingestion of valerian extracts as compared to the morning after ingestion of benzodiazepines where there was impairment of vigilance.

A study in Japan on the psychotropic effects of Japanese valerian root extract found that it acts on the central nervous system and may be an antidepressant.

A study in the United Kingdom found that valerian may be beneficial to health by reducing physiological reactivity during stressful situations.

Homeopathy

Homeopathy is a medical practice that uses extremely dilute plant or mineral substances, which have no side effects. Some individual homeopathic medicines can be prescribed for acute conditions such as aconite, which is specific for fear and terror. However, for symptoms of depression it is often more beneficial for the individual to see a homeopath to give a detailed history for prescription of the specific remedy for his or her case.

A study in France showed that aconite proved to be effective for children's postoperative agitation with 95 percent good results.

Hypnosis

An article in the *American Journal of Clinical Hypnosis*

summarized aspects of effective psychotherapy for major depression and described how hypnosis is helpful in reducing common symptoms of major depression such as agitation and rumination and thereby may decrease a client's sense of helplessness and hopelessness. It stated that hypnosis is also effective in facilitating the learning of new skills, a core component of all empirically supported treatments for major depression.

A study in India found that hypnosis combined with a later follow-up period of self-hypnosis, removed chronic repeated episodes of stress related hemoptysis in a 24-year-old patient.

Inositol

Inositol is a member of the vitamin B family.

A study in Israel compared inositol, a natural isomer of glucose, with an established drug, fluvoxamine, in the treatment of panic disorders. Inositol reduced a greater number of attacks per week and proved attractive in patients because it is a natural compound with few known side effects.

A second study in Israel found that inositol was effective as sole therapy for depression, and proved as effective as impramine in treating panic disorder.

Laughter

A team in Japan found that natural killer cell activity (NKCA) elevation and NKCA before and after a comic film seem to be related with the experiential aspects of laughter rather than with the expressive aspects.

Light Therapy

A study at Yale University found that morning light therapy has an antidepressant effect during pregnancy.

In Vancouver researchers found that an active bright

white light condition significantly reduced depression and premenstrual tension during symptomatic luteal phase in women with late luteal phase dysphoric disorder (LLPDD)

Seasonal affective disorder (SAD) is the name given to people who get depressed when they don't get enough natural sunlight.

A study in Sweden found that light therapy with concomitant and continued SSRI (citalopram) treatment is a useful strategy to achieve beneficial long-term effects in patients with seasonal affective disorder (SAD).

A study in Finland indicated that bright light administered twice a week, alone or combined with physical exercise, seemed to be a useful intervention for relieving seasonal mood slumps.

A study in the Netherlands demonstrated that bright light therapy had a positive effect on motor restless behavior in patients with dementia.

Magnetic Stimulation

Our heart and brain emit the most electromagnetism in the body. The heart's energy is measured by the electrocardiogram, and the brain's energy is measured by the electroencephalogram. Knowing the electromagnetic potential of the brain, many researchers have tried to manufacture devices to try to "balance" the brain's electromagnetic output. The following is a series of studies that show the benefit of such intervention.

A study in Chicago compared repetitive transcranial magnetic stimulation (rTMS), a noninvasive technique to modulate cortical excitability, to electroconvulsive therapy (ECT) in severely ill, depressed patients and found comparable therapeutic effects.

An article in the American Journal of Psychiatry reviews studies of "slow" rTMS and finds slow rTMS offers a new method for probing and possibly treating brain hyperexcitability syndromes.

In the U.K. another review of studies of the effectiveness of rTMS indicated its demonstratable beneficial effects in the treatment of depression.

A study in Iowa found that rTMS improved significantly the cognitive flexibility and conceptual tracking of middle-aged and elderly patients with refractory depression.

In Germany a report was published that described the treatment of a patient with major depression who had been hospitalized for 60 months during a period of seven years with no improvement, even from electroconvulsive therapy, but once treated with rTMS was discharged after just four weeks of daily treatment.

Meditation

Prayer, self-reflection, chanting, and meditation all have a soothing and calming effect on the psyche.

A study in Philadelphia concluded that a group mindfulness meditation training program can enhance functional status and well-being and reduce physical symptoms and psychological distress in a heterogeneous patient population, and that the intervention may have long-term beneficial effects as well.

A study in Canada found that a mindfulness meditation-based stress reduction program was effective in decreasing mood disturbance and stress symptoms in both male and female patients with a wide variety of cancer diagnoses, stages of illness, and ages.

Another study in Arizona investigated the short-term effects of an eight-week meditation-based stress reduction intervention on premedical and medical students and found that participation in the intervention could reduce self-reported state and trait anxiety, reduce reports of overall psychological distress including depression, increase scores on overall empathy levels, and increase scores on a measure of spiritual experiences at the termination of the intervention.

Melatonin

Melatonin is a hormone produced by the pineal gland and is responsible for our sleeping/waking cycle. It is elevated at night before bedtime and lowest in the morning. It has become a common sleep aid. By helping people get a good night's rest, it can lesson symptoms of anxiety and depression.

A pilot study in Argentina suggested that melatonin can be an alternative and safe treatment for patients with fibromyalgia. Adverse events were mild and transient.

Benzodiazepines are the most frequently used drug for the treatment of insomnia. However, prolonged use of benzodiazepine therapy is not recommended. A study in Israel found that controlled-release melatonin effectively facilitated discontinuation of benzodiazepine therapy while maintaining good sleep quality.

Mind-Body Medicine

The field of psychoneuroimmunology is successfully bridging the mind-body split in light of recent research that finds brain neurotransmitters and their effects in the gut and throughout the whole lymphatic system. This means our gut and, in effect, our whole body, can experience moods, which may be expressed as physical symptoms but are a direct effect of a shift in our emotions.

A review published in *Gerontology* found that there was significant impact of affective disorders on immune functions in the elderly subjects. Due to the high frequency in the aged of autoimmune, infectious, and neoplastic diseases it recommended a focus on the psychoneuroimmune interactions in old age.

A study in Ohio found that production of proto-inflammatory cytokines that influence conditions associated with aging can be directly stimulated by negative emotions and stressful experiences. Additionally, negative emotions also contributed to prolonged infection and delayed wound healing, processes that fuel sustained pro-inflammatory cytokine production.

A review conducted in Australia found that a number of studies have demonstrated that stress increase the risk of viral infection, and stress and depression can depress immunity whereas stress reduction can enhance immunity.

A study in South Africa found that acute phase proteins were significantly raised in a group of patients with depressive disorder and suggested there was an interaction between psychological state and immune system operative in host defenses.

An article in *Semin Clin Neuropsychiatry* reviewed evidence that showed a bi-directional relationship between the brain and the immune system. These findings implicated a role for the immune system in the cause of behavioral disorders in a wide range of medical illnesses.

A study in Japan investigated the relationship between the psychological and immunological state in patients with atopic dermatitis and found that patients with atopic dermatitis were significantly more depressive and scored higher for state anxiety. The study concluded that the psychological state is related to the immunological state.

A second study in Japan reports that recent psychoneuroimmunological research demonstrates that depression and other types of emotional stress damages the immune system, which can induce some physical diseases, especially for the elderly, who have weakened cell-mediated immune function and are more susceptible to influence by the damaged immune function caused by such psychiatric disfunction.

Appendix for Alternative Health Studies

In San Francisco, a review of clinical trials of mind-body-medicine (MBM) therapies are effective in improving quality of life, anxiety, and pain intensity for a variety of conditions.

Music Therapy

It was after both world wars that music therapy gained prominence as local musicians were hired by hospitals to play for shell-shocked soldiers. The response to music by anxious and depressed patients has been well documented over the years.

An article in the Intensive Crit Care Nurs discusses a study in which patients waiting for their cardiac catheterization benefitted from music therapy. Anxiety and heightened physiological values elicited by the stress response were reduced. Results also suggested that women waiting for cardiac catheterization experience a higher level of anxiety than males.

A study in Italy found that proctological patients who listened to a guided tour imagery tape and relaxing text before, during, and after surgery experienced reduced pain following anorectal surgery and improved quality of sleep.

In Norway an overview of central areas of application of music in clinical medicine found music has been used successfully to treat anxiety and depression and improve function in schizophrenia and autism. The supportive role of music has a natural field of application in palliative medicine and terminal care.

Phototherapy

A study in France found that phototherapy has been a successful alternative to medication, in addition to anti-depressive medication, and as a primary treatment of seasonal depression.

Psychodrama

Psychodrama is a form of therapy where patients act out scenarios of life events that give them insight into their problems.

A study in Massachusetts found that psychodrama groups with traumatized middle-school girls revealed significant decreases in group participants' self-reported difficulties in withdrawn behavior and anxiety/depression.

A review of three trials in the United Kingdom found that psychological intervention in the form of psychodynamic psychotherapy may be useful in the treatment of non-ulcer dyspepsia.

Reiki

Reiki is a form of bodywork that is actually an ancient natural healing art patterned after the healings performed by Jesus. Reiki uses a laying on of hands system of touch healing. It promotes healing on all levels: physical, mental, emotional, and spiritual.

An article in the Journal of Indian Medical Association has outlined the contemporary application of Reiki principles to the physical response to stress and stress related illnesses.

Religion

Dr. Larry Dossy has written a book, *The Power of Prayer*, citing volumes of research that prove the power of prayer to heal both physical and emotional imbalance.

A review of studies published in the International Journal of Psychiatry in Medicine found that if religious beliefs and practices improve coping, reduce stress, prevent or facilitate the resolution of depression, improve social support, promote healthy behaviors, and prevent alcohol and drug abuse, then a plausible mechanism exists by which physical health may be affected.

Reminiscence Therapy

A study in North Carolina demonstrated that reminiscence therapy is an effective means of reducing depression among institutionalized, rural-dwelling elders, especially older women, who resist treatment from mental health services for a variety of different reasons.

Therapeutic Touch

Therapeutic touch is defined as the sharing of life force energies between two or more people with the intent of causing a healing transformation physically and spiritually. It involves light touching to direct healing energy.

A study in Alabama found that therapeutic touch (TT), an intervention in which human energies are therapeutically manipulated, versus sham TT could produce greater pain relief as an adjunct to narcotic analgesia, produced a greater reduction in anxiety, and alterations in plasma T-lymphocyte concentrations among burn patients.

A study in Quebec, Canada, showed that TT treatments increased the sensation of well-being and reduced the depression and anxiety in persons with terminal cancer.

A study in New York State found that five postpartum women who participated in therapeutic touch during home visits for two months experienced many positive emotions.

An article in the Journal of Holistic Nursing discussed the beneficial effects of TT on seven hospitalized, adolescent psychiatric patients who received a total of 31 TT treatments over two two-week periods.

Thermal Therapy

A study in Italy showed that data on females and males with no psychiatric history, attending thermal facilities while testing for their psychoneurotic profiles, supported the hypothesis that a particular form of neurosis, in particular gastrointestinal referred somatic disease, may play a significant role in motivating request of thermal therapies.

Vitamins

A study in California on the effect of thiamin (vitamin B1) supplementation proved positive for nonspecific conditions such as anorexia, weight loss, fatigue, sleep disorders, and depression in an elderly Irish population with marginal thiamin deficiency.

In New York State 24 chronic schizophrenic patients were treated successfully with the addition of acetazolamide and thiamine to their unchanged existing therapies.

A study in Germany examined whether patients with Alzheimer's disease (AD) with subnormal vitamin B12 levels show more frequent behavioral and psychological symptoms of dementia than AD patients with normal vitamin B12 levels. The results show vitamin B12 could play a role in the pathogenesis of behavioral changes in AD.

• REFERENCES •

CHAPTER TWO

1. Szabo, Liz, *U.S.A. Today.* September 30, 2009; http://www.usatoday.com/news/health/2009-09-30-drug-overdose_N.htm
2. Vedantum S. *Washington Post.* January 9, 2002; page a01.
3. Vedantum S. *Washington Post.* May 21, 2002; Page A01.
4. Ann Landers website.
5. Screening for Mental Health, Inc. website.
6. Nintendo Neurology. *Scientific American*, August 2000.

CHAPTER THREE

1. Turner E.H., et al. "Selective publication of antidepressant trials and its influence on apparent efficacy." *New England Journal of Medicine.* 2008 358: 252-260.
2. *The Hoax of Learning and Behavior Disorders*, Citizens Commission on Human Rights (pamphlet), Los Angeles, 2001.

3. Zito, Julie Magno, "Trends in the Prescribing of Psychotropic Medications to Preschoolers," *Journal of the American Medical Association,* Feb 23, 2000, Vol. 283, No 8, pp. 1025-30.

4. West, Jean, "Children's drug is more potent that cocaine," *The Observer,* London, Sept 9, 2001.

5. Graham, J.E., et al., "A Double-blind, randomized, placebo-controlled trial of fluoxetine in children and adolescents with depression." *Arch. Gen. Psychiatry,* 1997; 54: 1031-37.

6. Breggin, Peter R., "Today's Kids Suffer Legal Drug Abuse," *Newsday,* Sept. 23, 1999, p.A53.

7. Gary Null interview with Dr. Fred Baughman, Feb 12, 2001.

8. DeGrandpre, Richard, *Ritalin Nation*, W.W. Norton & Co,. New York 1999, p. 160

9. Elkind, David, *The Hurried Child*, Addison-Wesley, New York, 1981.

10. Suriano, Robyn, "As Kids Get Put on Pills, Critics Fret," *Orlando Sentinel,* Nov. 26, 2001.

11. Gary Null interview with Dr. David Stein, Feb. 13, 2001.

12. *Ibid.*

13. Suriano, *op. cit.*

14. Harris, Gardiner, "Use of Mood-Altering Drugs to Control Toddler's Behavior Jumped in the '90's," *Wall Street Journal*, Feb. 23, 2000.

15. Robison, Holly, "Generation RX," *Parents,* Nov. 2001, p. 82.

16. Kaiser, David, "Commentary: Against Biologic Psychiatry," *Psychiatric Times*, CME Inc., *webmaster@mhsource.com.*

17. O'Meara, Kelly Patricia, "Writing May Be on the Wall for Ritalin," *Insight,* Oct. 16, 2000, omeara@insight.com

18. Zernike, Kate, and Melody Peterson, "Schools' Backing of Behavior Drugs Comes Under Fire," *The New York Times,* Aug. 19, 2001.

19. Breggin, Peter R., *Talking Back to Ritalin: What Doctors Aren't Telling You About Stimulants for Children,* Common Courage Press, Monroe, ME, 1998, p.5.

20. Lipkin, P.H., et. al., "Tics and dyskinesias associated with stimulant treatment in attention-deficit hyperactivity disorder." *Arch. Pediatr. Adolesc. Med.,* Aug. 1994, 148(8): 859-61.

21. Gerlach, J., et. al. "Methylphenidate, amorphine, THIP, and diazepam in monkeys. . . dopamine-GABA behavior related to psychoses and tardive dyskinesia," *Psychopharmacology (Berl.),* 1984, 82(1-2): 131-4.

22. Weiner, W.J., et al., "Methyphenidate-induced chorea: case report and pharmacological implications," *Neurology,* Oct. 1978, 28(10): 1041-4.

23. Young, J.G. "Methylphenidate-induced hallucinosis: case histories and possible mechanisms of action," *J. Dev. Behav. Pediatr.,* June 1981, 2(2): 35-8.

24. Silver, Larry B., *Dr. Larry Silver's Advice to Parents on Attention-Deficit Hyperactivity Disorder,* American Psychiatric Press, Washington D.C., 1993, p. 189.

25. Taylor, John F., *Helping Your Hyperactive/Attention Deficit Child,* Prima Publishing, Rocklin, Ca, 1994, p. 87.

26. Sears, William, and Lynda Thompson, *The A.D.D. Book: New Understandings, New Approaches to Parenting Your Child*. Little, Brown and Co., New York, 1998 p. 235.
27. Swanson, J.S., et al., "Stimulant Medication and the Treatment of Children with Attention Deficit Disorder: A review of Reviews," *Exceptional Children*, 1993, Vol. 60, pp. 154-61.
28. Gary Null interview with Janet Hall, Feb. 13, 2001.
29. *Ibid.*
30. Associated Press, "Ritalin Maker Sued Over Girl's Death," *The Record* (New Jersey), Jan 9, 2000, p. A-3.
31. Gary Null interview with Dr. Dragovic, Feb. 13, 2001.
32. *Ibid.*
33. Wang, G.J., et. al., "Methylphenidate decreases regional cerebral blood flow in normal human subjects," *Life Sci.*, 1994, 54(9): PL143-6.
34. Suplee, Curt, "Brain not finished developing by age 6, scientists now say," *The Philadelphia Inquirer*, Mar. 9, 2000.
35. Henderson, T.A., and Fischer, V.W., "Effects of methylphenidate (Ritalin) on mammalian myocardial ultrastructure," *American Journal of Cardiovascular Pathology*, 1995, 5(1):68-78.
36. DeGrandepre, *op. cit.*
37. *Ibid.*, p.19.
38. Zernike, Kate, and Melody Peterson, "Schools' Backing of Behavior Drugs Comes Under Fire," *The New York Times*, Aug. 19, 2001.

References

39. Ziegler, Nicole, "Recreational Ritalin," The Associated Press, abcNEWS.com, May 5, 2000.

40. Clerman, G., ed., *Contemporary Directions in Psychopathology,* 1986.

41. Cauchon, Dennis, "Patients often aren't informed of full danger," *USA Today,* Dec. 6 1995.

42. Boodman, Sandra G., "Shock Therapy. . . It's Back," *The Washington Post,* Sept. 24, 1996, p. Z14.

43. Boodman, *op. cit.*

44. *Electroshock as Head Injury: Report for the National Head Injury Foundation,* Sept. 1991.

45. Samant, Sydney, *Clinical Psychiatry News,* Mar. 1983.

46. Freeman, C., and Kendall, R., "Patients' experience of and attitudes to electroconvulsive therapy," *Annals of the New York Academy of Sciences,* 462 (1986), 341-52.

47. Gerring, Joan P., and Shields, Helen M., "the Identification and Management of patients with high risk for cardiac arrhythmias during modified ECT, "*J. Clin. Psychiatry,* 43-4.

48. Appendix to Breeding, John, "Electroshock." Based on an article in the *J. Of Humanistic Psychology,* Winter 2000, Vol. 40, No. 1, pp. 65-69, citing Ali, P.B., and Tidmarsh., M.D., Cardiac Rupture During Electroconvusive Therapy Anesthesia 1997; 52: 884-895.

49. Boodman, *op. cit.*

50. Edelson, E., "ECT elicits controversy-and results," *Houston Chronicle,* Dec. 28, 1988, p.3 as reported in "Electroshock; Death, Brain Damage,

Memory Loss, and Brainwashing," op. cit., p.493.

51. Opton, EM., Jr., Letter to the members of the panel, National Institutes of Health Consensus Development Conference on Electroconvulsive Therapy, June 4, 1985, as cited in Frank, L.R., "Electroshock; death, brain damage, memory loss, and brainwashing," op. Cit., p. 497.

52. Boodman, SG., "Shock therapy... it's back," op cit.

53. Cauchon, Dennis, "Patients often aren't informed of full danger," op. cit.

54. Frank, LR., "Electroshock; death, brain damage, memory loss, and brainwashing," op. cit., p.494.

55. Ibid.

56. Viscoit, D., *The Making of a Psychiatrist*. Greenwich, CT, Faucett, 1972, in Leonard Roy Frank, "Electroshock; Death ..." op. cit., p.494

CHAPTER FOUR

1. Baker, S.L., "A Nation on Mind Altering Drugs: Antidepressants Most Commonly Prescribed Drugs in the U.S." NaturalNews with Columbia University Medical Center and New York State Psychiatric Institute, New York. Sept 8, 2009. http://www.naturalnews.com/027054_drugs_antidepressants_health.html

2. *Journal of the American Medical Association*, August 2001.

3. *The New England Journal of Medicine*, Feb 14, 2002, pp.498-SOS, 524-531.

4. Boseley S, Scandal of scientists who take money for papers ghostwritten by drug companies, *The Guardian*, February 7, 2002.

References

5. Is academic medicine for sale?, 342(20), *N Engl J Med* May 18, 2000, pp. 1516-8.
6. Postapproval Risks 1976-1985, GAO/PEMD 90-15 FDA Drug Review, p.3.
7. "Drugmaker Upset; New book attacks popular antidepressant Prozac," Associated Press, April 6, 2000.
8. Glenmullen J, *Prozac Backlash*.
9. Kramer P, *Listening to Prozac*.
10. Breggin, Peter R, M.D., *Your Drug May Be Your Problem; How and Why to Stop Taking Psychiatric Medications*, Perseus Books, 1999.
11. Breggin, Peter R, M.D., *Talking Back to Ritalin, Revised ; What Doctors Aren't Telling You About Stimulants and ADHD*, Perseus Books, 2001.
12. Breggin, Peter R, M.D., *Toxic Psychiatry; Why therapy, empathy, and love must replace the drugs, electroshock, and biochemical theories of the "new psychiatry."* St. Martin's Press, 1994.
13. Breggin, Peter R, M.D., *The Anti-Depressant Fact Book; What Your Doctor Won't Tell You About Prozac, Zoloft, Paxil, Celexa and Luvox*.
14. Breggin, Peter R, M.D., *Talking Back to Prozac; What doctors aren't telling you about today's most controversial drug*, St. Martin's Press, 1995.
15. Breggin, Peter R, M.D., *Brain-Disabling Treatments in Psychiatry: Drugs, Electroshock, and the Role of the FDA*, Springer Publishing Co., 1997.
16. http://www.breggin.com/
17. Breggin, Peter B, M.D., *Electroshock; Its Brain-Disabling Effects*, Springer Publishing Company, 1979.

18. Mansbridge P, CBC News and Current Affairs, Jun 12, 2001.
19. "Paxil Maker Ordered to Pay $8 Million," The Associated Press, June 6, 2002.
20. Wang PN, Liao SQ, Liu RS, Liu CY, Chao HT, Lu SR, Yu HY, Wang SJ, Liu HC, Effects of estrogen on cognition, mood, and cerebral blood flow in Alzheimer's Disease; a controlled study, 54(11) *Neurology*, June 13, 2000, pp.206 I-6.
21. Breuer B, Martucci C, Wallenstein 5, Likourezos A, Libow LS, Peterson A, Zumoff B, Relationship of endogenous levels of sex hormones to cognition and depression in frail, elderly women, 10(3) *Am J Geriatr Psychiatry*, May 2002, Pp.311-20.
22. Campbell M, Silva RR, Kafantaris V, Locascio JJ, Gonzalez NM, Lee D, Lynch NS, Predictors of side effects associated with lithium administration in children, 27(3) *Psychopharmacol Bull.*, 1991, pp.373-SO.
23. Silva RR, Campbell M, Golden RR, Small AM, Pataki CS, Rosenberg CR, Side effects associated with lithium and placebo administration in aggressive children, 28(3) *Psychopharmacol Bull.*, 1992, pp.319-26.
24. Malone RP, Delaney MA, Luebbert JF, Cater J, Campbell M, A double-blind placebo-controlled study of lithium in hospitalized aggressive children and adolescents with conduct disorder, 57(7) *Arch Gen Psychiatry*, July 2000, pp.649-54.
25. Mavissakalian M, Perel J, Goo S, Specific side effects of long-term imipramine management of panic disorder, 22(2) *J Clin Psychopharmacol*, Apr 2002, pp.155-61.

26. Holt WL, van Iperen CE, Schrijver G, Bartelink AK, Severe hyponatremia during therapy with fluoxetine, 156(6) *Arch Intern Med.*, Mar 25, 1996, pp.681-2.

27. Girault C, Richard JC, Chevron V, Goulle JP, Droy JM, Bonmarcliand G, Leroy J, Syndrome of inappropriate secretion of antidiuretic hormone in two elderly women with elevated serum fluoxetine, 35(1) *J Toxicol Clin Toxicol*, 1997, pp.93-5.

28. Burke D, Fanker 5, Fluoxetine and the syndrome of inappropriate secretion of antidiuretic hormone (SIADH), 30(2) *Aust N Z J Psychiatry*, Apr 1996, pp.29 S-8.

29. Bourguignon RP, Dangers of fluoxetine, 349(9046) *Lancet*, Jan 18, 1997, p.24.

30. Braun D, Nippert B, Loeuille D, Blain H, Trechot P, Interstitial pneumopathy induced by fluoxetine, 20(10) *Rev Med Interne*, Oct 1999, PP.949-50.

31. Martinez Ortiz JJ, Hyperthyroidism secondary to antidepressive treatment with fluoxetine, 16(11) *An Med Interna*, Nov 1999, pp.583-4.

32. Bates GD, Khin-Maung-Zaw F., Movement disorder with fluoxetine, 37(1) *J Am Acad Child Adolesc Psychiatry*, Jan 1998, pp. 14-5.

33. Wilmshurst PT, Kumar AV, Subhyaloid hemorrhage with fluoxetine, 10(Pt 1) Eye, 1996, p.141.

34. Michael A, Mayer C, Fluoxetine-induced anaesthesia of vagina and nipples, 176 *Br J Psychiatry*, Mar 2000, P.299.

35. Hwang AS, Magraw RM, Syndrome of inappropriate secretion of antidiuretic hormone due to fluoxetine, 146(3) *Am J Psychiatry*, Mar 1989, p.399.

36. Anand KS, Prasad A, Pradhan SC, Biswas A, Fluoxetine-induced tremors, 47(6) *J Assoc Physicians India*, June 1999, pp.651-2.

37. Cohen BJ, Mahelsky M, Adler L, More cases of SIADH with fluoxetine, 147(7) *Am J Psychiatry*, July 1990, pp.948-9.

38. Vishwanath BM, Navalgund AA, Cusano W, Navalgund KA, Fluoxetine as a cause of SIADH, 148(4) *Am J Psychiatry*, April 1991, pp.542-3.

39. Buchman N, Strous RD, Baruch Y, Side effects 0f long-term treatment with fluoxetine, 25(1) *Clin Neuropharmacol*, Jan 2002, pp.SS-7.

40. Stanford JA, Currier TD, Gerhardt GA, Acute locomotor effects of fluoxetine, sertraline, and nomifensine in young versus aged Fischcr 344 rats, 71(1-2) *Pharmacol Biochem Behav*, Jan-Feb 2002, pp.325-32.

41. Rothschild AJ, Sexual side effects of antidepressants, 61 Suppl 11 *J Gun Psychiatry,* 2000, pp.28-36.

42. Baton R, Yeragani VK, Pohi R, Ramesh C, Sexual dysfunction during antidepressant treatment, 54(6) *J Clin Psychiatry*, June 1993, pp.209-12.

43. Opbroek A, Delgado PL, Laukes C, McGahuey C, Katsanis J, Moreno FA, Manber R, Emotional blunting associated with SSRI-induced sexual dysfunction. Do SSRIs inhibit emotional responses?, 5(2) *Tnt J Neuropsychopharmacol*, June 2002, pp.147-51.

44. Murray JB, Physiological mechanisms of sexual dysfunction side effects associated with antidepressant medication, 132(4) *J Psychol*, July 1998, pp.407-16.

45. Woodrum ST, Brown CS, Management of SSRI-induced sexual dysfunction, 32(11) *Ann Pharmacother*, Nov 1998, pp. 1209-15.

46. Sproule BA, Naranjo CA, Brenmer KE, Hassan PC, Selective serotonin reuptake inhibitors and CNS drug interactions. A critical review of the evidence, 33(6) *Clin Pharmacokinet*, Dec 1997, pp.454-71.

47. Bozikas V, Petrikis F, Karavatos A, Urinary retention caused after fluoxetinerisperidone combination, 15(2) *J Psychopharmacol*, June 2001, pp. 142-3.

48. Fava M, Rankin M, Sexual functioning and SSRIs, 63 Suppl 5 *J Clin Psychiatry*, 2002, pp. 13-6.

49. Bagdy G, Graf M, Anheuer ZE, Modos EA, Kantor S, Anxiety-like effects induced by acute fluoxetine, sertraline or m-CPP treatment are reversed by pretreatment with the 5-HT2C receptor antagonist SB-242084 but not the 5-HT IA receptor antagonist WAY-100635, 4(4) *Tnt J Neuropsychopharmaco*, Dec 2001, pp,399-408.

50. Nurnberg HG, Lauriello J, Hensley PL, Parker LM, Keith SJ, Sildenafil for iatrogenic serotonergic antidepressant medication-induced sexual dysfunction in 4 patients, 60(1) *J Clin Psychiatry*, Jan 1999, pp.33-5.

51. Tollefson GD, Sayler ME, Course of psychomotor agitation during pharmacotherapy of depression: analysis from double-blind controlled trials with fluoxetine, 4(6) *Depress Anxiety*, 1996, pp.294-311.

57. Reichenberg-Ullman J, Homeopathy: a highly effective alternative to antidepressants (for

treatment of mental depression), Townsend Letter for Doctors and Patients, April 2001.

58. Montgomery SA, Judge R, Treatment of depression with associated anxiety: comparisons of tricyclic antidepressants and selective serotonin reuptake inhibitors, 403 *Acta Psychiatr Scand Suppl*, 2000, pp.9-16.

59. Cook BL, Helms PM, Smith RE, Tsai M, Unipolar depression in the elderly. Reoccurrence on discontinuation of tricyclic antidepressants, 10(2) *J Affect Disord*, Mar 1986, pp.91-4.

60. Graber MA, Weckmann M, Pharmaceutical company internet sites as sources of information about antidepressant medications, 16(6) *CNS Drugs*, 2002, pp.419-23.

61. Anderson JL, The immune system and major depression, 6(2) *Adv Neuroimmunol*, 1996, pp. 119-29.

62. Macs M, Vandoolaeghe E, Ranjan R, Bosmans E, Bergmans R, Desnyder R, Increased serum interleukin-1--receptor-antagonist concentrations in major depression, 36(1-2) *J Affect Disorder*, Dec 24, 1995, pp.29-36.

63. Elgun S, Keskinege A, Kumbasar H, Dipeptidyl peptidase IV and adenosine deaminase activity. Decrease in depression, 24(8) *Psychoneuroendocrinology*, Nov 1999, pp.823-32.

64. Irwin M, Psychoneuroimmunology of depression; clinical implications, 16(1) *Brain Behav Immun*, Feb 2002, pp. 1-16.

65. Hese RT, Gruszczynski W, Szwed A, Kielc M, Zalitacz M, Comparative studies of adverse effects in patients with refractory depression treated

with amitryptyline, mianserin and unilateral ECT, 35(2) *Psychiatr Pol*, Mar-Apr 2001, pp. 219-29.

66. Clayton AH, Pradko JF, Croft HA, Montano CB, Leadhetter RA, BoldenWatson C, Bass KI, Donahue RM, Jamerson BD, Metz A., Prevalence of sexual dysfunction among newer antidepressants, 63(4) *J Clin Psychiatry*, Apr 2002, pp.357-66.

67. Lemmo Walter, Unraveling antidepressant medications: what you & your physician may not know, Townsend Letter for Doctors and Patients, July 2001.

68. Covelli V, Maffione AB, Nacci C, Tato E., Jirillo E, Stress, neuropsychiatric disorders and immunological effects exerted by benzodiazepines, 20(2) *Immunopharmacol Immunotoxicol*, May 1998, pp. 199-209.

69. Kupfer DJ, Pathophysiology and management of insomnia during depression, 11(4) *Ann Clin Psychiatry*, Dec 1999, pp.267-76.

70. Miller NS, Gold MS, Benzodiazepines: a major problem. Introduction, 8(1-2) *J Subst Abuse Treat*, 1991, pp.3-7.

71. Juergens SM, Benzodiazepines and addiction, 16(1) *Psychiatr Clin North Am*, March 1993, pp.75-86.

72. Holden J, Benzodiazepine dependence, 233(1478) *Practitioner*, Nov 8, 1989, pp. 1479-80, 1483.

73. Bernik MA, Scares MB, Scares CN, Benzodiazepines: patterns of use, tolerance and dependence, 48(1) *Arq Neuropsiquiatr*, Mar 1990, pp. 131-7.

74. Olivier H, Fitz-Gerald MJ, Babiak B., Benzodiaz-

epines revisited, 150(10) *J La State Med Soc*, Oct 1998, pp.483-5.

75. Kuribara H, Kishi E, Maruyama Y, Does dihydrohonokiol, a potent anxiolytic compound, result in the development of benzodiazepine-like side effects?, 52(8) 1 *Pharm Pharmacol,* Aug 2000, pp.1017-22.

76. Pettinati HM, Stephens SM, Willis KM, Robin SE, Evidence for less improvement in depression in patients taking benzodiazepines during unilateral ECT, 147(8) *Am J Psychiatry*, Aug 1990, 1029-35.

77. Simmer ED, A fugue-like state associated with diazepam use, 164(6) *Mil Mcd*, June 1999, pp.442-3.

78. Engel WR, Grau A, Inappropriate secretion of antidiuretic hormone associated with lorazepam, 297(6652) *BMJ*, Oct 11988, p.858.

79. Loo H, Olie JP, Poirier MF, Amado I, Psychotropic Drugs and Behavior, 56(2) *Ann Pharm Fr,* 1998, pp.75-82.

80. Paterniti S, Dufouil C, Alperovitch A., Long-term benzodiazepine use and cognitive decline in the elderly; the Epidemiology of Vascular Aging Study, 22(3) *J Clin Psychopharmacol,* Jun 2002, pp.285-93.

81. Pigott TA, Seay SM, A review of the efficacy of selective serotonin reuptake inhibitors in obsessive-compulsive disorder, 60(2) *J Clin Psychiatry*, Feb 1999, pp.101-16.

82. Papakostas Y, Stefanis C, Sinouri A, Trikkas G, Papadimitriou G, Pittoulis S., Increases in prolactin levels following bilateral and unilateral

ECT, 141(12) *Am J Psychiatry*, Dec 1984, pp. 1623-4.

83. Markowitz JS, Kellner CH, DeVane CL, Beale MD, Folk J, Burns C, Liston HL, Intranasal sumatriptan in post-ECT headache: results of an open-label trial, 17(4) *J ECT*, Dec 2001, pp.280-3.

84. Brodaty H, 1-lickie I, Mason C, Prenter L, A prospective follow-up study of ECT outcome in older depressed patients, 60(2) *J Affect Disord*, Nov 2000, pp. 101-1 1.

85. Fromm-Auch D, Comparison of unilateral and bilateral ECT. evidence for selective memory impairment, 141. *Br J Psychiatry*, Dec 1982, pp.608-1 3.

86. Squire LR, Zouzounis JA, ECT and memory: brief pulse versus sine wave, 143(5), *Am J Psychiatry*, May 1986, pp. 596-601.

87. Pettinati HM, Rosenberg J, Memory self-ratings before and after electroconvulsive therapy: depression-versus ECT induced, 19(4) *Biol Psychiatry*, Apr 1984, pp.539-48.

88. Calev A, Nigal D, Shapira B, Tubi N, Chazan S, Ben-Yehuda Y, Kugelmass 5, Lerer B, Early and long-term effects of electroconvulsive therapy and depression on memory and other cognitive functions, 179(9) *J Nerv Ment Dis*, Sep 1991, pp.526-33.

89. Squire LB, Chace PM, Slater PC, Retrograde amnesia following electroconvulsive therapy, 260(5554) *Nature*, Apr 29, 1976, pp.775.

90. Frith CD, Stevens M, Johnstone EC, Deakin JF, Lawler P, Crow TJ, Effects of ECT and

depression on various aspects of memory, 142 *Br J Psychiatry*, June 1983, PP.61 0-7.

91. McAllister DA, Perri MG, Jordan RC, Rauscher FP, Sattin A, Effects of ECT given two vs. three times weekly, 21(1) *Psychiatry Res*, May 1987, pp.63-9.

92. Stewart C, Jeffery K, Reid 1, LTP-like synaptic efficacy changes following electroconvulsive stimulation, 5(9) *Neuroreport*, May 9, 1994, pp. 1041-4.

93. CalevA, Cohen R, Tubi N, Nigal D, Shapira B, Kugelmass S, Lerer B, Disorientation and Bilateral Moderately Suprathreshold Titrated ECT, 7(2) *Convuls Ther* 1991, pp.99-1 10.

94. Neylan TC, Canick JD, Hall SE, Reus VI, Sapoisky RM, Wolkowitz OM, Cortisol levels predict cognitive impairment induced by electroconvulsive therapy, 50(5) *Biol Psychiatry*, Sep 1, 2001, Pp.331-6.

95. Tang WK, Ungvari GS, Asystole during electroconvulsive therapy: a case report, 35(3) *Aust N ZJ Psychiatry*, Jun 2001, pp.382-5.

96. Ng C, Schweitzer I, Alexopoulos P, Celi E, Wong L, Tuck-well V, Sergejew A, Tiller J, Efficacy and cognitive effects of right unilateral electroconvulsive therapy, 16(4)] *ECT*, Dec 2000, pp.370-9.

97. Dubovsky SL, Buzan R, Thomas M, Kassner C, Cullum CM, Nicardipine improves the antidepressant action of ECT but does not improve cognition, 17(1)] *ECT*, Mar 2001, pp. 3-10.

98. Rao V, Lyketsos CG, The benefits and risks of ECT for patients with primary dementia who also suffer from depression, 15(8) *mt J Geriatr*

Psychiatry, Aug 2000, pp.729-35.

99. Lisanby SH, Maddox JH, Prudic J, Devanand DP, Sackeim HA, The effects of electroconvulsive therapy on memory of autobiographical and public events, 57(6) *Arch Gen Psychiatry*, Jun 2000, pp.58 1-90.

100. Shapira B, Tubi N, Lerer B, Balancing speed of response to ECT in major depression and adverse cognitive effects: role of treatment schedule, 16(2) *J ECT*, Jun 2000, Pp.97-109.

101. Sackeim HA, Luber B, Moeller JR Prudic J, Devanand DP, Nobler MS, Electrophysiological correlates of the adverse cognitive effects of electroconvulsive therapy, 16(2)] *ECT,* Jun 2000, pp. 110-20.

102. Squire LR, Slater PC, Miller PL, Retrograde amnesia and bilateral electro convulsive therapy. Long-term follow-up, 38(1) *Arch Gen Psychiatry,* Jan 1981, pp.89-95.

103. Shellenberger W, Miller MJ, Small IF, Milstein V, Stout JR, Follow-up study of memory deficits after ECT, 27(4) Can J Psychiatry, Jun 1982, pp. 32 5-9.

104. Sobin C, Sackeim HA, Prudic .J, Devanand DP, Moody BJ, McElhiney MC, Predictors of retrograde amnesia following ECT, 152(7) *Am J Psychiatry*, Jul 1995, pp.995-1001.

105. Weiner RD, Retrograde amnesia with electroconvulsive therapy: characteristics and implications, 57(6) *Arch Gen Psychiatry,* Jun 2000, pp.591-2.

106. Rosenberg, Pettinati HM, Differential memory complaints after bilateral and unilateral ECT, 141(9) *Am J Psychiatry*, Sep 1984, pp. 1071-4.

CHAPTER FIVE

1. Epidemiology of medical error. Weingart, SN. et al. *BMJ*. 2000;320: 774-777 (18 March).

2. Reporting and preventing medical mishaps: lessons from non-medical near miss reporting systems. Barach, P. and Small S. *BMJ*. 2000;320:759-763 (18 March).

3. The scandal of poor medical research. Altman, DG. *BMJ* 1994; 308:283-284 (29 January).

4. Sponsored drug trials show more-favourable outcomes. Wahlbeck K, et al. *BMJ*. 1999;318:464 (13 February).

5. Physicians and the Pharmaceutical Industry: Is a Gift Ever Just a Gift? Wazana, A. *JAMA*. 2000;283:373-380.

6. Reasons for not seeing drug representatives. Griffith D. *BMJ* 1999;319: 69-70 (10 July).

7. Medical societies accused of being beholden to the drugs industry. Gottlieb S. *BMJ* 1999;319:1321 (20 November).

8. "Routine" preoperative studies. Which studies in which patients? Marcello PW, Roberts PL. *Surg Gun North Am* 1996 Feb;76(1):1 1-23.

9. Value of routine preoperative chest x-rays: a meta-analysis. Archer C, Levy AR, McGregor M. *Can J Anaesth* 1993 Nov;40(1 1):1022-7.

10. Accuracy of fecal occult blood screening for colorectal neoplasia A prospective study using Hemoccult and HemoQuant tests. Ahlquist DA, et al. *JAMA*. 1993 Mar 10;269(10):1262-7.

11. Consumption of NSAIDs and the development of congestive heart failure in elderly patients:

an underrecognized public health problem. Page J, Henry D. *Arch Intern Med.* 2000 Mar 27;160(6):777-84.

12. Study throws doubt on protective effects of HRT for heart disease. Gottlieb S. *BMJ* 2000;320:826 (25 March).

13. Impact of postmenopausal hormone therapy on cardiovascular events and cancer: pooled data from clinical trials. Elina Hemminki, et al. *BMJ* 1997;315:149-153 (19 July).

14. Mortality associated with oral contraceptive use 25 year follow up of cohort of 46 000 women from Royal College of General Practitioners' oral contraception study. Beral V, et al. *BMJ* 1999;318:96-100 (9 January).

15. Oral contraceptives and fatal pulmonary embolism, Parkin L, Skegg DCG, Wilson M, Herbison GP, Paul C. *Lancet.* 2000; 355: 2088,2133-2134.

16. Ovarian tumors in a cohort of infertile women. Bossing MA, Daling JR, Weiss NS, Moore DE, Self SG. *N Engl J Med.* 1994 Sep 22;331(12): 771-6.

17. Rates of Cesarean delivery--United States, 1993. *MMWR Moth Mortal Wkly Rep.* 1995 Apr 21;44(15):303-7.

18. Cesarean section: medical benefits and costs. Shearer EL. *Soc Sci Med.* 1993 Nov;37(10):1223-31.

19. Drug use and pulmonary death rates in increasingly symptomatic asthma patients in the UK. Meier CR; Jick H. *Thorax.* 52(7):612-7 1997 Jul

20. Adverse effects of inhaled corticosteroids. Hanania NA; Chapman KR; Kesten S. *Am J Med.* 98(2):196-208 1995 Feb.

21. Cancer undefeated. Bailar JC 3rd; Gornik HL. *N Engl J Med.* 336(22):1569-74 1997 May 29.

22. Gallbladder carcinoma: a 28 year experience. Frezza EE, Mezghebe H. *Int Surg.* 1997 Jul-Sep;82(3):295.300.

23. Pathological prognostic factors in the second British Stomach Cancer Group trial of adjuvant therapy in resectable gastric cancer, Yu CC; et al. *J Cancer.* 71(5):1106-10 1995 May.

24. Pre-operative radiotherapy prolongs survival in operable esophageal carcinoma: a randomized, multicenter study of pre-operative radiotherapy and chemotherapy. The second Scandinavian trial in esophageal cancer. Nygaard K; et al. *World J Surg,* 16(6):1 104-9; discussion 1110 1992 Nov-Dec. 25a.

25. Lack of evidence for a role of chemotherapy in the routine management of locally advanced head and neck cancer, Tannock IF; Browman G. *J Gun Oncol.* 4(7):1121-6 1986 Jul.

26. Outcome of combination chemotherapy in extensive stage small-cell lung cancer: any treatment related progress? Lassen UN, Hirsch FR, Osterlind.

27. K, Bergman B, Dombernowsky P. *Lung Cancer* 1998 Jun;20(3):15160.

28. Interferon alfa-2a and interleukin-2 with or without cisplatin in metastatic melanoma: a randomized trial of the European Organization for Research and Treatment of Cancer Melanoma Cooperative Group. Keilholz U; et al. *J Clin Oncol,* 15(7):2579._88 1997 Jul.

29. Randomized study of 5-FU and CCNU in pancre-

atic cancer. Report of the Veterans Administration Surgical Adjuvant Cancer Chemotherapy Study Group. Frey C; Twomey P; Keehn R; Elliott D; Higgins C. *Cancer*, 47(1):27-31 1981 Jan 1.

30. Failure of cytotoxic chemotherapy, 1983-1988, and the emerging role of monoclonal antibodies for renal cancer. Yagoda A; Bander NH. *Urol Int*, 44(6):338-45 1989.

31. Late effects of radiation therapy for cancer of the uterine cervix. Zippin C; Lum D; Kohn HI; Bailar JC 3rd. *Cancer Detect Prev*, 4(1-4):487-92 1981.

32. Intensive blood-glucose control with sulphonylureas or insulin compared with conventional treatment and risk of complications in patients with type 2 diabetes (UKPDS 33). UK Prospective Diabetes Study (UKPDS) Group. *Lancet*. 1998 Sep 12;352(9131):83753

33. Controversies in Management: Case for early treatment is not established. Chadwick, D. *BMJ* 1995;310:177-178 (21 January).

34. Notice to Readers: Fourth Decennial International Conference on Nosocomial and Healthcare-Associated Infections. *MMWR*. February 25, 2000 /49(07);138.

CONCLUSION

1. Luo H, Meng F, Jia Y, Zhao X. Clinical research on the therapeutic effect of the electro-acupuncture treatment in patients with depression. *Psychiatry Clin Neurosci*. 1998 Dec;52 Suppl:S338-40.

2. Roschke J, Wolf C, Muller MJ, Wagner P, Mann

K, Grozinger M, Bech S.The benefit from whole body acupuncture in major depression. *J Affect Disord*. 2000 Jan-Mar;57(I -3):73-8 1.

3. Knight B, Mudge C, Openshaw S, White A, Hart A.Effect of acupuncture on nausea of pregnancy: a randomized, controlled trial. *Obstet Gynecol*. 2001 Feb;97(2):184-8.

4. Eich H, Agelink MW, Lehmann E, Lemmer W, Klieser F. Acupuncture in patients with minor depressive episodes and generalized anxiety. Results of an experimental study. *Fortschr Neurol Psychiatr*. 2000 Mar;68(3): 13-7-44.

5. Bullock ML, Kiresuk TJ, Sherman RE, Lenz SK, Culliton PD, Boucher TA, Nolan C. A large randomized placebo controlled study of auricular acupuncture for alcohol dependence. *J Subst Abuse Treat*. 2002 Mar; 220:71-7.

6. Russell AL, McCarty MR DL-phenylalanine markedly potentiates opiate analgesia; an example of nutrient/pharmaceutical up-regulation of the endogenous analgesia system. *Med Hypotheses*. 2000 Oct;55(4):283-8.

7. Ernst F. A primer 0f complementary and alternative medicine commonly used by cancer patients. *Med J Aust*. 2001 Jan 15; 1 74(2):88-92.

8. Manber R, Allen JJ, Morris MM. Alternative treatments for depression: empirical support and relevance to women. *J Clin Psychiatry*. 2002 Jul;63 (7) :628-40.

9. Dello Buono M, Urciuoli 0, Marietta P, Padoani W, De Leo D. Alternative medicine in a sample of 655 community-dwelling elderly. *J Psychosom Res*. 2001 Mar;50(3):147-54.

10. Ernst F. A primer of complementary and alternative medicine commonly used by cancer patients. *Med J Aust.* 2001 Jan 15;174(2):88-92.

11. D'Elia G, Hanson L, Raotma H. L-tryptophan and 5-hydroxytryptophan in the treatment of depression, a review. *Acta Psychiatr Scand.* 1978 Mar;57(3):239-52.

12. Lam RW, Zis AP, Grewal A, Delgado PL, Charney DS, Krystal JH. Effects of rapid tryptophan depletion in patients with seasonal affective disorder in remission after light therapy. *Arch Gen Psychiatry.* 1996 Jan;53(l):41-4.

13. Abou-Saleh MT, Ghubash R, Karim L, Krymski M, Anderson DN. The role of pterins and related factors in the biology of early postpartum depression. *Eur Neuropsychopharmacol.* 1999 Jun;9(4):295-300.

14. Spillrnann MK, Van der Does AJ, Rankin MA, Vuolo RD, Alpert JE, Nierenberg AA, Rosenbaum JF, Hayden D, Schoenfeld D, Fava M. Tryptophan depletion in SSRI-recovered depressed outpatients. *Psychopharmacology (Ben).* 2001 May;155(2):123-7.

15. Blokland A, Lieben C, Deutz NE. Anxiogenic and depressive-like effects, but no cognitive deficits, after repeated moderate tryptophan depletion in the rat. *J Psychopharmacol.* 2002 Mar; 16(1):39-49.

16. Young SN, Leyton M. The role of serotonin in human mood and social interaction. Insight from altered tryptophan levels. *Pharmacol Biochem. Behav.* 2002 Apr;71(4):857-65.

17. Khalsa DS. Integrated medicine and the preven-

tion and reversal of memory loss. *Altern Then Health Med.* (1998 Nov) 4(6):38-43.

18. Holmes C, Hopkins V, Hensford C, MacLaughlin V, Wilkinson D, Rosenvrnge H. Lavender oil as a treatment for agitated behaviour in severe dementia: a placebo controlled study. *Int J Geriatr Psychiatry.* 2002 Apr;1 7(4):305-8.

19. Dunn C, Sleep J, Collett D. Sensing an improvement: an experimental study to evaluate the use of aromatherapy, massage and periods of rest in an intensive care unit. *J Ad Nurs.* 1995 Jan;21(1):34-40.

20. Burns E, Blarney C, Ersser S, Lloyd AJ, Barnetson L. The use of aromatherapy in intrapartum midwifery practice an observational study. *Complement Then Nurs Midwifery.* 2000 Feb;6(l):33-4.

21. Buckle J. The role of aromatherapy in nursing care. *Nurs Gun North Am.* 2001 Mar;36(1):57-72.

22. Lee KG, Mitchell A, Shibamoto T. Antioxidative activities of aroma extracts isolated from natural plants. *Biofactors.* 2000;13(1-4):173_8.

23. Chattacharya SK, Battacharya A, Sairam K, Ghosal S. Anxiolyticantidepressant activity of Withania somnifera glycowithanolides: an experimental study. *Phytomedicine.* 2000 Dec;7(6):463-9.

24. Bhattacharya SK, Battacharya A, Chakrabarti A. Adaptogenic activity of Siotone, a polyherbal formulation of Ayurvedic rasayanas. *Indian J Exp Biol.* 2000 Feb;38(2):119-28.

25. Jaiswal AK, Bhattacharya SK, Acharya SB. Anxiolytic activity of Azadirachta indica leaf extract in rats. *Indian J Exp Biol.* 1994 Jul;32(7):489-91.

26. Long L, Huntley A, Ernst E. Which complemen-

tary and alternative therapies benefit which conditions? A survey of the opinions of 223 professional organizations. *Complement Ther Med.* 2001 Sep;9(3) 178-85.

27. Saeki Y. The effect of foot-bath with or without the essential oil of lavender on the autonomic nervous system: a randomized trial. *Complement Ther Med.* 2000 Mar;8(1):2-7.

28. Rastelli A, Sartori A, Ferrari G. Arsenic-iron balneotherapy in anxiety syndromes. Controlled clinical study at the Levico thermal baths. *Minerva Med.* 1985 Dec 22;76(49-50):2291-301.

29. Evcik D, Kizilay B, Gokcen F. The effects of balneotherapy on fibromyalgia patients. *Rheumatol Int.* 2002 Jun;22(2): 56-9.

30. Armijo Valenzuela M. Spa therapy and sadness. *An R Acad Nac Med (Madr).* 1999;116(2):279-95.

31. Buskila D, Abu-Shakra M, Neumann L, Odes L, Shneider E, Flusser D, Sukenik S. Balneotherapy for fibromyalgia at the Dead Sea. *Rheumatol Int.* 2001 Apr;20(3):105-8.

32. Wright J, Glum GA, Roodman A, Febbraro GA. A bibliotherapy approach to relapse prevention in individuals with panic attacks. *J Anxiety Disord.* 2000 Sep-Oct;14(5):483-99.

33. Christensen H, Griffiths KM, Korten A. Web-based cognitive behavior therapy: analysis of site usage and changes in depression and anxiety scores. *J Med Internet Res.* 2002 Jan-Mar;4(l):e3.

34. Kupshik GA, Fisher CR. Assisted bibliotherapy: effective, efficient treatment for moderate anxiety problems. *Br J Gen Pract.* 1999 Jan;49(438):47-S.

35. Montgomery P. Media-based behavioural treat-

ments for behavioural disorders in children. *Cochrane Database Syst Rev.* 2001;(2):CD002206.

36. Pearistein T, Steiner M. Non-antidepressant treatment of premenstrual syndrome. *J Clin Psychiatry.* 2000;61 Suppl 12:22-7.

37. Bauman WA, Shaw S, Jayatilleke E, Spungen AM, Herbert V. Increased intake of calcium reverses vitamin B12 malabsorption induced by metformin. *Diabetes Care.* 2000 Sep;23(9):1227-31.

38. Mercola J. Low cholesterol causes aggressive behavior and depression. Townsend Letter for Doctors and Patients. 2001 May.

39. Heimberg RG. Cognitive-behavioral therapy for social anxiety disorder: current status and future directions. *Biol Psychiatry.* 2002 Jan 1;51(1):101-8.

40. Clark DB, Agras WS. The assessment and treatment 0f performance anxiety in musicians. *Am J Psychiatry.* 1991 May; 148(5):598-605.

41. Generalised anxiety disorder: treatment options. Sramek JJ, Zarotsky V Cutler NR. *Drugs.* 2002;62(11):1635-48.

42. Safren SA, Heimberg RG, Brown EJ, Holle C. Quality of life in social phobia. *Depress Anxiety.* 1996-97;4(3):126-33.

43. Pearlstein T, Steiner M. Non-antidepressant treatment of premenstrual syndrome. *J Clin Psychiatry.* 2000;61 Suppl 12:22-7.

44. Goisman RM, Warshaw MG, Keller MB. Psychosocial treatment prescriptions for generalized anxiety disorder, panic disorder, and social phobia, 1991-1996. *Am J Psychiatry.* 1999 Nov;156(11):1819-21.

45. Demeter E, Rihmer Z, Frecska E. Colour associations as predictors of the effectiveness of anti-depressant pharmacotherapy in endogenous depressive patients. *Psychopathology.* 1985;18(5-6):305-9.

46. de Craen AJ, Roos PJ, Leonard de Vries A, Kleijnen J. Effect of colour of drugs: systematic review of perceived effect of drugs and of their effectiveness. *BMJ.* 1996 Dec 21-28;313(7072):1624-6.

47. Coldwell SE, Getz T, Milgrom P, Prall CW, Spadafora A, Ramsay DS. CARL: a LabVIEW 3 computer program for conducting exposure therapy for the treatment of dental injection fear. *Behav Res Ther.* 1998 Apr;36(4):429-41.

48. Ant W, Callies F, Allolio B. DHEA replacement in women with adrenal insufficiency-pharmacokinetics, bioconversion and clinical effects on well-being, sexuality and cognition. *Endocr Res.* 2000 Nov;26(4):505-11.

49. Cogan E. DHEA: orthodox or alternative medicine? *Rev Med Brux.* 2001 Sep;22(4):A381-6.

50. Young AH, Gallagher P, Porter RJ. Elevation of the cortisol-dehydroepiandrosterone ratio in drug-free depressed patients. *Am J Psychiatry.* 2002 Jul;159(7):123 7-9.

51. Goodyer IM, Herbert J, Tamplin A, Altham PM. First-episode major depression in adolescents. Affective, cognitive and endocrine characteristics of risk status and predictors of onset. *Br J Psychiatry.* 2000 Feb;176:142-9.

52. Nagata C, Shimizu H, Takami R, Hayashi M, Takeda N, Yasuda K. Serum concentrations of estradiol and dehydroepiandrosterone sulfate

and soy product intake in relation to psychologic well-being in pre- and postmenopausal Japanese women. *Metabolism.* 2000 Dec;49(12):1561-4.

53. Michael A, Jenaway A, Paykel ES, Herbert J. Altered salivary dehydroepiandrosterone levels in major depression in adults. *Biol Psychiatry.* 2000 Nov 15;48(10):989-95.

54. Fabian TJ, Dew MA, Pollock BG, Reynolds CF 3rd, Mulsant BH, Butters MA, Zmuda MD, Linares AM, Trottini M, Kroboth PD. Endogenous concentrations of DHEA and DHEA-S decrease with remission of depression in older adults. *Biol Psychiatry.* 2001 Nov 15;50(10):767-74.

55. Huppert FA, Van Niekerk JK, Herbert J. Dehydroepiandrosterone (DHEA) supplementation for cognition and well-being. *Cochrane Database Syst Rev.* 2000;(2):CD000304.

56. Cohen JH, Kristal AR, Neumark-Sztainaer D, Rock CL, Neuhouser ML. Psychological distress is associated with unhealthful dietary practices. *J Am Diet Assoc.* 2002 May; 102(5):699-703.

57. Balcombe NR, Ferry PC, Saweirs WM. Nutritional status and well being. Is there a relationship between body mass index and the well-being of older people. *Curr Med Res Opin.* 2001;17(1):1-7.

58. Schmidt MH, Mocks F, Lay B, Eisert HC, Fojkar R, Fritz-Sigmund D, Marcus A, Musaeus B. Does oligoantigenic diet influence hyperactive conduct-disordered children, a controlled trial. *Eur Child Adolesc Psychiatry.* 1997 Jun;6(2):88-95.

59. Vatn MH. Food intolerance and psychosomatic experience. *Scand J Work Environ Health.* 1997;23 Suppl 3:75-8.

60. Rogers PJ. A healthy body, a healthy mind: long-term impact of diet on mood and cognitive function. *Proc Nutr Soc.* 2001 Feb;60(l):13543.

61. Breakey J. The role of diet and behaviour in childhood. *J Pediatr Child Health.* 1997 Jun;33(3):190-4.

62. Bittman BB, Berk LS, Felten DL, Westengard J, Simonton OC, Pappas J, Ninehouser M. Composite effects of group drumming music therapy on modulation of neuroendocrine-immune parameters in normal subjects. *Altern Ther Health Med.* 2001 Jan;7(l):38-47.

63. Horrobin DF. The role of essential fatty acids and prostaglandins in the premenstrual syndrome. *J Reprod Med.* 1983 Jul;28(7):465-8.

64. Stoll AL, Severus WE, Freeman MP, Rueter 5, Zboyan HA, Diamond E, Cress KK, Marangell LB. Omega 3 fatty acids in bipolar disorder: a preliminary double-blind, placebo-controlled trial. *Arch Gen Psychiatry.* 1999 May;56(5):407-12.

65. Rudin DO. The major psychoses and neuroses as omega-3 essential fatty acid deficiency syndrome: substrate pellagra. *Biol Psychiatry.* 1981 Sep;16(9):837-S0.

66. Mischoulon D, Fava M. Docosahexanoic acid and omega-3 fatty acids in depression. *Psychiatr Clin North Am.* 2000 Dec;23(4):785-94.

67. Martinsen EW. Physical activity for mental health. *Tidsskr Nor Laegeforen.* 2000 Oct 20;120(25):3054_6.

68. Jorm AF, Christensen H, Criffiths KM, Rodgers B. Effectiveness of complementary and self-help treatments for depression. *Med J Aust.* 2002 May

20;176 Suppl:S84-96.

69. Castro CM, Wilcox 5, O'Sullivan P, Baumarin K, King AC. An exercise program for women who are caring for relatives with dementia. *Psychosom Med.* 2002 May-Jun;64(3):458_68.

70. Paladini AC, Marder M, Viola H, Wolfman C, Wasowski C, Medina JH. Flavonoids and the central nervous system: from forgotten factors to potent anxiolytic compounds. *J Pharm Pharmascoi.* 1999 May;5 1(5) :519-26.

71. Viola H, Wolfman C, Levi de Stein M, Wasowski C, Pena C, Medina JH, Paladini AC. Isolation of pharmacologically active benzodiazepine receptor ligands from Tilia tomentosa (Tiliaceae). *J Ethnopharmacol.* 1994 Aug; 44(1):47_53.

72. Butterweck V, Nishibe 5, Sasaki T, Uchida M. Antidepressant effects of apocynum venetum leaves in a forced swimming test. *Biol Pharm Bull.* 2001 Jul;24(7):848-5 1.

73. Gaby A. Can depressed people benefit from folic acid supplementation? Townsend Letter for Doctors and Patients. 2001 Jan.

74. Thompson MB, Coppens NM. The effects of guided imagery on anxiety levels and movement of clients undergoing magnetic resonance imaging. *Holist Nurs Pract.* 1994 Jan;8(2):59-69

75. Holden-Lun C. Effects of relaxation with guided imagery on surgical stress and wound healing. *Res Nurs Health.* 1988 Aug;11(4):23 5-44,

76. Speck BJ. The effect of guided imagery upon first semester nursing students performing their first injections. *J Nurs Educ.* 1990 Oct;29(8) 346-50.

77. Ilouldin AD, McCorkle B, Lowery BJ. Relaxation

training and psychoimmunological status of bereaved spouses. A pilot study. *Cancer Nurs.* 1993 Feb;16(l):47-52

78. McKinney CH, Antoni MH, Kumar M, Tims FC, McCabe PM. Effects of guided imagery and music (CIM) therapy on mood and cortisol in healthy adults. *Health Psychol.* 1997 Jul;16(4):390-400.

79. Rees BL. Effect of relaxation with guided imagery on anxiety, depression, and self-esteem in primiparas. *J Holist Nurs.* 1995 Sep;13(3):255-67.

80. Eller LS. Guided imagery interventions for symptom management. *Anna Rev Nurs Res.* 1999;17:57-84.

81. Burns DS. The effect of the bonny method of guided imagery and music on the mood and life quality of cancer patients. *J Music Ther.* 2001 Spring;38(1) 51-65.

82. Leja AM. Using guided imagery to combat postsurgical depression. *J Gerontol Nurs.* 1989 Apr;1 5(4):7-11.

83. Liske E, Hanggi W, Henneicke-von Zepelin HH, Boblitz N, Wustenberg P, Rahlfs VW. Physiological investigation of a unique extract 0f black cohosh (Cimieifugae racemosae rhizoma): a 6-month clinical study demonstrates no systemic estrogenic effect, *J Womens Health Gend Based Med.* 2002 Mar; 1 l(2):163-74.

84. Satyan KS, Jaiswal AK, Ghosal S Bhattacharya SK. Anxiolytic activity of ginkgolic acid conjugates from Indian Ginkgo biloba. *Psychopharmacology (Ben)* 1998 Mar; 136(2):148-52.

85. Bradwejn J, Zhou Y, Koszycki D, Shlik J. A double-blind, placebo-controlled study on the effects

of Gotu Kola (Centella asiatica) on acoustic startle response in healthy subjects. *J Clin Psychopharmacol.* 2000 Dec 20(6) :680-4.

86. Malseh U, Kieser M. Efficacy of kava-kava in the treatment of non psychotic anxiety, following pretreatment with benzodiazepines. *Psychopharmacology (Ben).* 2001 Sep;157(3):27783.

87. Watkins LL, Connor KM, Davidson JR. Effect of kava extract on vagal cardiac control in generalized anxiety disorder: preliminary findings. *J Psychopharmucol.* 2001 Dec;lS(4):2836.

88. Wheatley D. Kava and valerian in the treatment of stress-induced insomnia. *Phytother Res.* 2001 Sep;l 5(6):549-5 1.

89. Pittler MH, Edzard E. Kava extract for treating anxiety. *Cochrane Database Syst Rev.* 2001;(4):CD003383.

90. Grunze H, Langosch J, Schirrmacher K, Bingmann D, Von Wegerer J, Walden J. Kava pyrones exert effects on neuronal transmission and transmembraneous cation currents similar to established mood stabilizers-a review. *Prog Neuropsychopharmacol Biol Psychiatry.* 2001 Nov;25(8): 1555-70.

91. Gerhard U, Linnenbrink N, Georghiadou C, Hobi V.Vigilance decreasing effects of 2 plant-derived sedatives. *Schweiz Rundsch Med Prax.* 1996 Apr 9;850 5):473-81.

92. Sakamoto T, Mitani Y, Nakajima K. Psychotropic effects of Japanese valerian root extract. *Chem Pharm Bull (Tokyo).* 1992 Mar;40(3):758_6l.

93. Cropley M, Cave Z, Ellis J, Middleton RW. Effect of kava and valerian on human physiologi-

cal and psychological responses to mental stress assessed under laboratory conditions. *Phytother Res.* 2002 Feb; 16(1) :23-7.

94. Alibeu JP, Jobert J. Aconite in homeopathic relief of post-operative pain and agitation in children. *Pediatnie.* 1990;45(7-8):465-6.

95. Yapko M. Hypnosis in treating symptoms and risk factors of major depression. *Am J Clin Hypn.* 2001 Oct;44(2):97-108.

96. Palan BM, Lakhani JD. Converting the "threat" into a "challenge": a ease of stress-related hemoptysis managed with hypnosis. *Am J Clin Hypn.* 1991 Apr;33(4):241-7.

97. Gruzelier J, Smith F, Nagy A, Henderson D. Cellular and Immoral immunity, mood and exam stress: the influences of self-hypnosis and personality predictors. *J Psychophysiol.* 2001 Aug;42 (1):55-71.

98. Palatnik A, Frolov K, Fwt M, Benjamin J. Double-blind, controlled, crossover trial of inositol versus fluvoxamine for the treatment of panic disorder. *J Clin Psychopharmacol,* 2001 Jun;21(3):335-9.

99. Benjamin J, Agam G, Levine J, Bersudsky Y, Kofman O, Belmaker RH. Inositol treatment in psychiatry. *Psychopharmacol Bull.* 1995;31(1): 167-75.

100. Takahashi K, Iwase M, Yamashita K, Tatsumoto Y, Ue H, Kuratsune H, Shimizu A, Takeda M. The elevation of natural killer cell activity induced by laughter in a crossover designed study. *Int J Mol Med.* 2001 Dec ;8 (6) :645-50.

101. Oren DA, Wisner KL, Spinelli M, Epperson CN,

Peindl KS, Terman JS, Terman M. An open trial of morning light therapy for treatment of antepartum depression. *Am J Psychiatry.* 2002 Apr;159(4):666-9.

102. Lam RW, Carter D, Misri S, Kuan AJ, Yatham LN, Zis AP. A controlled study of light therapy in women with late luteal phase dysphorie disorder. *Psychiatry Res.* 1999 Jun 30;86(3):185_92.

103. Thorell LH, Kjellman B, Arned M, Lindwall-Sundel K, Walinder J, Wetterberg L. Light treatment of seasonal affective disorder in combination with citalopram or placebo with 1-year follow-up. *Gun Psychopharmacol.* 1999 May; 14 Suppl2:S7-ll.

104. Leppamalu SJ, Partonen IT, Hurme J, Hauki(a JK, Lonnqvist JK. Randomized trial of the efficacy of bright-light exposure and aerobic exercise on depressive symptoms and serum lipids. *J Curt Psychiatry.* 2002 Apr; 63(4)316-21.

105. Haffmans PM, Sival RC, Lucius SA, Cats Q, van Gelder L. Bright light therapy and melatonin in motor restless behaviour in dementia: a placebo-controlled study. *Int J Geriatr Psychiatry.* 2001 Jan; 16(l):106-10.

106. Janicak PG, Dowd SM, Martis B, Alam D, Beedle D, Krasuski J, Strong MJ, Sharma R, Rosen C, Viana M. Repetitive transcranial magnetic stimulation versus electroconvulsive therapy for major depression: preliminary results of a randomized trial. *Biol Psychiatry.* 2002 Apr 15;51(8):659-67.

107. Hoffman RE, Cavus I. Slow transcranial magnetic stimulation, long-term depotentiation, and brain hyperexcitability disorders. *Am J Psychia-*

try. 2002 Jul;159(7):1093-102.

108. McNamara B, Ray JL, Arthurs OJ, Boniface S.Transcranial magnetic stimulation for depression and other psychiatric disorders. *Psychol Med.* 2001 Oct;31(7):1141-6.

109. Moser DJ, Jorge RE, Manes F, Paradiso S, Benjamin ML, Robinson RG. Improved executive functioning following repetitive transcranial magnetic stimulation. *Neurology.* 2002 Apr 23;58(8);1288-90.

110. Smesny S, Volz HP, Liepert J, Tauber R, Hochstetter A, Sauer H.Repctitive transcranial magnetic stimulation (rTMS) in the acute and long-term therapy of refractory depression–a case report. *Nervencsrzt.* 2001 Sep; 72(9):734-8.

111. Reibel DK, Greeson JM, Brainard GC, Rosenzweig S. Mindfulness-based stress reduction and health-related quality of life in a heterogeneous patient population. *Gen Hosp Psychiatry.* 2001 Jul-Aug;23(4):183-92.

112. Speca M, Carlson LE, Goodey E, Angen M. A randomized, wait-list controlled clinical trial: the effect of a mindfulness meditation-based stress reduction program on mood and symptoms of stress in cancer outpatients. *Psychosom Med.* 2000 Sep-Oct;62(5):613-22.

113. Shapiro SL, Schwartz GE, Bonner G. Effects of mindfulness-based stress reduction on medical and premedical students. *J Behav Med.* 1998 Dec; 21 (6):581-99.

114. Citera G, Arias MA, Maldonado-Cocco JA, Lazaro MA, Rosemffet MG, Brusco LI, Schemes EJ, Cardinalli DP. The effect of melatonin in patients

with fibromyalgia: a pilot study. *Clin Rheumatol.* 2000;19(1):9-13.

115. Garfinkel D, Zisapel N, Wainstein J, Laudon M. Facilitation of benzodiazepine discontinuation by melatonin: a new clinical approach. *Arch Intern Med.* 1999 Nov 8; 159(20):2456-60.

116. Guidi L, Tricerri A, Frasca D, Vangeli M, Errani AR, Bartoloni C. Psychoneuroimmunology and aging. *Gerontology.* 1998;44(5):247-6

117. Kiecolt-Glaser JK, McGuire L, Robles TF, Glaser R. Emotions, morbidity, and mortality: new perspectives from psychoneuroimmunology. *Annu Rev Psychol.* 2002;53:83-107.

118. Sali A. Psychoneuroimmuriology. Fact or fiction? *Aust Pam Physician.* 1997 Nov;26(11):1291-4, 1296-9.

119. Berk M, Wadee AA, Kuschke RH, O'Neill-Kerr A. Acute phase proteins in major depression. *J Psychosom Res.* 1997 Nov;43(5):52934

120. Raison CL, Miller AH. The neuroimmunology of stress and depression. *Semin Clin Neuropsychiatry.* 2001 Oct;6(4):277_94.

121. Hashiro M, Okumura M. The relationship between the psychological and immunological state in patients with atopic dermatitis. *J Dermatol Sci.* 1998 Mar 16(3):231-5

122. Wada H. Problems and strategies in the treatment of mental disorders in elderly patients with physical illness. *Nippon Ronen Igakkai Zasshi* 2000 Nov; 37(1 1):885-8.

123. Barrows KA, Jacobs BP. Mind-body medicine: An introduction and review of the literature. *Med Clin North Am.* 2002 Jan;86(1): 11-31.

124. Hamel WJ. The effects of music intervention on anxiety in the patient waiting for cardiac catheterization. *Intensive Crit Care Nurs.* 2001 Oct;17(5):279-85,

125. Renzi C, Peticca L, Pescatori M. The use of relaxation techniques in the perioperative management of proctological patients: preliminary results. *Int J Colorectal Dis.* 2000 Nov;15(5-6):313-6.

126. Myskja A, Lindbaek M. Examples of the use of music in clinical medicine. *Tidsskr Nor Laegeforen.* 2000 Apr 10; 120(10):1186-90.

127. Metzger JY, Berthou V, Perrin P, Sichel JP. Phototherapy: clinical and therapeutic evaluation of a 2-year experience. *Encephale.* 1998 Sep-Oct; 24(5):480-5.

128. Carbonefi DM, Parteleno-Barehmm C. Psychodrama groups for girls coping with trauma. *Int J Group Psychother.* 1999 Jul;49(3):285-306.

129. Soo S, Moayyedi P, Decks J, Delaney B, Lewis M, Forman D. Psychological interventions for non-ulcer dyspepsia. *Cochrane Database Syst Rev.* 2001;(4): CD002301.

130. Satya AJ. Stress management for patient and physician. *J Indian Med Assoc.* 2001 Feb;99(2):90-2.

131. Koenig HG. Religion and medicine III: developing a theoretical model. *Int J Psychiatry Med.* 2001;31(2):199-216.

132. Jones ED, Beck-Little R. The use of reminiscence therapy for the treatment of depression in rural-dwelling older adults. *Issues Ment Health Nurs.* 2002 Apr; 23(3):279.-90.

133. Turner JG, Clark A, Gauthier DK, Williams

M. The effect of therapeutic touch on pain and anxiety in burn patients. *J Adv Nurs.* 1998 Jul;28(l):10-20.

134. Giasson M, Bouchard L. Effect of therapeutic touch on the well-being of persons with terminal cancer. *J Holist Nurs.* 1998 Sep;l6(3):383-98.

135. Kiernan J. The experience of Therapeutic Touch in the lives of five postpartum women. *MCN Am J Matern Child Nurs.* 2002 Jan-Feb;27(l):47-53.

136. Hughes PP, Meize-Grochowski R, Harris CN. Therapeutic touch with adolescent psychiatric patients. *J Holist Nurs.* 1996 Mar; 14(l):6-23.

137. Comazzi AM, Nielsen NP, Zizolfi 5, Dioguardi N. Neurotic and depressive status related to organic pathology in patients in thermal therapy. *Minerva Med.* 1991 Jul-Aug;82(7-8):463-75.

138. Smidt U, Cremin FM, Grivetti LE, Clifford A. Influence of thiamin supplementation on the health and general well-being of an elderly Irish population with marginal thiamin deficiency. *J Gerontol.* 1991 Jan;46(l): M16-22.

139. Sacks W, Esser AH, Feitel B, Abbott K. Acetazolamide and thiamine: an ancillary therapy for chronic mental illness. *Psychiatry Res.* 1989 Jun;28(3):279-88.

140. Meins W, Muller- fhomsen T, Meier-Baumgartner HP. Subnormal serum vitamin B12 and behavioural and psychological symptoms in Alzheimer's disease. *Int Geriatr Psychiatry.* 2000 May; 15(5):415-8.